# Cognitive Science and the Unconscious

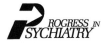PROGRESS IN PSYCHIATRY

*David Spiegel, M.D.*
*Series Editor*

# Cognitive Science and the Unconscious

*Edited by*
*Dan J. Stein, M.B.*

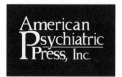

American Psychiatric Press, Inc.

Washington, DC
London, England

**Note:** The authors have worked to ensure that all information in this book concerning drug dosages, schedules, and routes of administration is accurate as of the time of publication and consistent with standards set by the U.S. Food and Drug Administration and the general medical community. As medical research and practice advance, however, therapeutic standards may change. For this reason and because human and mechanical errors sometimes occur, we recommend that readers follow the advice of a physician who is directly involved in their care or in the care of a member of their family.

Books published by the American Psychiatric Press, Inc., represent the views and opinions of the individual authors and do not necessarily represent the policies and opinions of the Press or the American Psychiatric Association.

Copyright © 1997 American Psychiatric Press, Inc.
ALL RIGHTS RESERVED
Manufactured in the United States of America on acid-free paper
First Edition   00   99   98   97     4   3   2   1

American Psychiatric Press, Inc.
1400 K Street, N.W., Washington, DC   20005

**Library of Congress Cataloging-in-Publication Data**
Cognitive science and the unconscious / edited by Dan J. Stein. — 1st ed.
      p.      cm. — (Progress in psychiatry series : #52)
      Includes bibliographical references and index.
      ISBN 0-88048-498-5 (alk. paper)
      1.   Psychoanalysis.   2.   Subconsciousness.   3.   Cognitive
science.   I.   Stein, Dan J.   II.   Series.
      [DNLM:   1.   Psychoanalytic Theory.   2.   Cognition.   3.   Un-
conscious (Psychology).      W1 PR6781L no.52 1997 / WM 460 C6765
1997]
   RC506.C56   1997
   616.89'17—dc20
   DNLM/DLC                                                     96-30885
   for Library of Congress                                          CIP

**British Library Cataloguing in Publication Data**
A CIP record is available from the British Library.

*For Heather, Gabriella, and Joshua*

# Contents

# Contributors

**Marylene Cloitre, Ph.D.**
Director of Psychology, Payne Whitney Clinic, New York, New York

**Ralph Hoffman, M.D.**
Associate Professor of Psychiatry, Yale Psychiatric Institute, New Haven, Connecticut

**Mardi J. Horowitz, M.D.**
Professor of Psychiatry and Director, Program on Conscious and Unconscious Mental Processes, University of California, San Francisco

**Howard S. Kurtzman, Ph.D.**
Chief, Cognitive Science Program, National Institute of Mental Health, Rockville, Maryland

**George Lakoff, Ph.D.**
Professor of Linguistics, University of California, Berkeley, California

**David Li, M.D.**
University of California–San Francisco Medical Center, San Francisco, California

**David Spiegel, M.D.**
Professor of Psychiatry and Behavioral Sciences and Director, Psychosocial Treatment Laboratory, Stanford University School of Medicine, Stanford, California

**Dan J. Stein, M.B.**
Director of Research, Department of Psychiatry, University of Stellenbosch, Tygerberg, South Africa

**Joel Weinberger, Ph.D.**
Clinical psychologist, researcher, and associate professor,
Derner Institute for Advanced Psychological Studies,
Adelphi University, Garden City, New York

**Joshua Weiss, Ph.D.**
Clinical psychologist, researcher, and assistant professor,
Bar-Ilan University, Ramat Gan, Israel

**Jeffrey E. Young, Ph.D.**
Director, Cognitive Therapy Center, New York, New York

# Introduction to the Progress in Psychiatry Series

The Progress in Psychiatry Series is designed to capture in print the excitement that comes from assembling a diverse group of experts from various locations to examine in detail the newest information about a developing aspect of psychiatry. This series emerged as a collaboration between the American Psychiatric Association's (APA) Scientific Program Committee and the American Psychiatric Press, Inc. Great interest is generated by a number of the symposia presented each year at the APA annual meeting, and we realized that much of the information presented there, carefully assembled by people who are deeply immersed in a given area, would unfortunately not appear together in print. The symposia sessions at the annual meetings provide an unusual opportunity for experts who otherwise might not meet on the same platform to share their diverse viewpoints for a period of 3 hours. Some new themes are repeatedly reinforced and gain credence, whereas in other instances disagreements emerge, enabling the audience and now the reader to reach informed decisions about new directions in the field. The Progress in Psychiatry Series allows us to publish and capture some of the best of the symposia and thus provide an in-depth treatment of specific areas that might not otherwise be presented in broader review formats.

Psychiatry is, by nature, an interface discipline, combining the study of mind and brain, of individual and social environments, of the humane and the scientific. Therefore, progress in the field is rarely linear—it often comes from unexpected sources. Furthermore, new developments emerge from an array of viewpoints that do not necessarily provide immediate agreement but rather expert examination of the issues. We intend to present innovative ideas and data that will enable you, the reader, to participate in this process.

We believe the Progress in Psychiatry Series will provide you with an opportunity to review timely, new information in specific fields of interest as they are developing. We hope you find that the excitement of the presentations is captured in the written word and that this book proves to be informative and enjoyable reading.

David Spiegel, M.D.
Series Editor
Progress in Psychiatry Series

# Foreword

Howard S. Kurtzman, Ph.D.

Everyone relies on some notion of an unconscious. But these notions vary in content and degree of elaboration. What is needed is a scientific investigation of the unconscious that will identify its essential characteristics. While such a research effort has been under way for over a century, the work of the last decade has been especially rigorous and imaginative. The present volume surveys a major strand of this new research: the formulation and testing of psychodynamic claims—stemming from Janet as well as Freud—using the approaches of contemporary cognitive science. The ultimate goal of this work is the integration of psychodynamic and cognitive theory.

This, of course, is not the first time that a linkage between psychodynamics and cognition has been attempted. In the 1940s and 1950s, John Dollard, Neal Miller, and their colleagues sought to assimilate various Freudian ideas into then-current neobehaviorist learning theory. Dollard and Miller were aware of the limitations of that era's learning theory and did try to extend it, at least schematically, toward what would eventually become full-fledged cognitive theory. Their work was widely praised and contained lasting insights, but its direct influence on subsequent research was limited. Arguably, though, it did much to create the atmosphere for later advances, including not only the lines of research represented in this book but also the formulation of behavioral and cognitive therapies.

Working during that same period on the psychoanalytic side, David Rapaport and other ego psychologists argued for understanding dynamic mechanisms in terms of the perceptual, memory, and reasoning capacities described by experimental psychologists. In fact, although rarely acknowledged in histories of cognitive science, the psychodynamic emphasis on mental representations and active cognitive processes was one of the factors contributing to the emergence of cognitive approaches out of behaviorism. Rapaport and his colleagues made only limited progress, but various contemporary psychoanalysts, including Marshall Edelson and Philip Holzman, have continued the call for the integration of psychoanalytic and cognitive concepts.

Most of the researchers now exploring the interface of cognition and psychodynamics come from a clinical background rather than from cognitive science. In general, cognitive scientists know little about psychodynamics, beyond an oversimplified Freud, and many are hostile toward it. However, this situation is likely to change as the rigorous work represented by this volume becomes better known among cognitive scientists. In fact, researchers working in social cognition, a subfield of cognitive science pursued mainly by experimental psychologists, have already shown increased interest in psychodynamic mechanisms. Their adaptation of psychodynamics points toward a more profound understanding of cognition and its relations with personality and social interaction. This, in turn, may lead to the enrichment of clinical theory and practice.

Progress in clinical work is important because current cognitive-behavioral therapies and psychopharmacological treatments are not fully satisfactory across all patients. Unconscious patterns and conflicts do seem to be at the root of certain patients' difficulties, and so psychodynamic approaches are warranted. Within some recent trends in cognitive-behavioral therapy, dynamic mechanisms, including conflictual and other interactive processes, have been posited. While it is premature to say that cognitive-behavioral and psychodynamic approaches are converging, they are surely moving closer together. By linking cognitive and psychodynamic perspectives on the unconscious at the basic science level, the work in this volume provides a foundation for further interaction of these perspectives at the clinical level. Integrationist therapists such as Paul Wachtel (who was a student of Dollard) have pro-

moted just such efforts. Indeed, some topics of primary importance within both basic and clinical work—for example, the mu-
tual influences of affect and thought, the recovered/false memory
issue—can be adequately investigated only from a dual cognitive
and psychodynamic perspective.

A difficulty of carrying out research in this area is that cognitive
science and psychodynamics each offer a number of concepts of
the unconscious. For the most part, these varied concepts are not
contradictory but rather address different aspects or levels of
analysis of the unconscious. Nonetheless, organizing the concepts
into an overall theoretical structure will be a challenge, especially
when concepts from one of the fields must be connected to those
in the other. Researchers from one field must become sufficiently
educated in the other field to understand fully the sources and
implications of its concepts.

Although a worthy ideal, complete convergence or integration
of cognitive and psychodynamic approaches is not necessary for
their interaction to produce valuable insights. One need not even
accept all the major assumptions and claims of the fields to make
use of portions of their results. Perhaps, then, the greatest significance of the research in this volume is that, in the attempt to
integrate the two fields, it tests the limits of and indicates new
directions for each of them.

# Chapter 1

# Introduction: Cognitive Science and the Unconscious

Dan J. Stein, M.B.

## Rationale for This Volume

"I have chosen to write a book about cognitive science because I consider this area to be the most exciting new line of inquiry undertaken by scientists in the past few decades."

Howard Gardner (1985, p. 7)

"The concept of the unconscious has long been knocking at the gates of psychology and asking to be let in."

Sigmund Freud (1938/1963, p. 223)

The notion of the unconscious lies at the heart of psychoanalytic theory and psychodynamic therapy. It would be difficult to overestimate the enormous effect that this construct has had on psychiatric theory and practice in the last century. Indeed, there are some who would argue that the notion of the unconscious has revolutionized our way of thinking about the world. It has been said that Copernicus showed that the Earth was not at the center of the universe, Darwin demonstrated that humanity was only one of a number of evolving species, and Freud added to this de-centering process by indicating that conscious, rational thought was not the most significant characteristic of humankind (Bhaskar 1978).

Nevertheless, psychoanalytic notions of the unconscious have received more than a little criticism. Psychoanalysis has been accused of failing to meet the standards of scientific thought and

1

practice, of devising explanations that are impossible to falsify, and of lacking an adequate experimental basis (Grunbaum 1993). Indeed, much about the notion of the psychodynamic unconscious is at odds with modern science. When Freud speaks of the laws of psychic energetics, the modern neurobiologist is lost. Similarly, when a modern psychoanalyst such as Kernberg talks about, say, unconscious projection of part-objects, the academic psychologist who demands operational definitions and laboratory methodologies can only shake his or her head in dismay (Widiger 1994).

Of course, academic psychology has had its own problems. The behaviorist emphasis on stimulus-response models has rightly been criticized as an inadequate basis for a science of human mind. This approach was barely interested in consciousness, much less the unconscious (although there were a number of exceptions, including the work of Dollard and Miller [1950], wherein a courageous effort was made to tackle psychodynamic constructs). The theorist interested in the unconscious would therefore seem to have few adequate choices, being faced with either a rich but outmoded psychoanalytic literature or a precise but irrelevant behaviorist approach.

Over the last few decades, however, academic psychology has witnessed a dramatic revolution with the emergence of a cognitive paradigm. The multidisciplinary field of cognitive science has become firmly established as a new and fruitful way of understanding the mind (Baars 1986; Gardner 1985). Although dissatisfaction with the behavioral approach was an important factor in the cognitive revolution, perhaps equally important was the emergence of computational science and concomitant computational models of the mind. Such computational models allow new approaches to thinking about the mind—approaches that include both conscious and unconscious processing—and can be taken to be the defining feature of cognitive science.

In contrast to psychoanalysis, cognitive science has firm roots in the laboratory and relatively little basis in the clinic. Although cognitive-behavioral therapy has drawn on the constructs of cognitive science, it remains a relatively independent endeavor. For the clinician, the rigorous laboratory methodologies of cognitivist approaches to the unconscious may appear dry and dull in comparison with the complexity and richness of clinical material. "The Unconscious" of psychoanalysis becomes the more mundane "unconscious processing" of cognitive science. The rich context of a particular patient may be lost in laboratory investigation of a series of normal subjects, and the clinical relevance of the cognitivist approach may seem unclear.

The crucial question arises, then, of whether a worthwhile exchange can be set up between cognitive and clinical science. A steady interchange of theory and method between cognitive and clinical science has in fact proceeded in recent years (Stein 1992a, 1994). This intersection appears to hold promise for the development of a dialogue that combines the theoretical clarity and empirical rigor of cognitive science with the richness and complexity of clinical work. Such a dialogue may provide a basis for theoretical and therapeutic integration within psychiatry in general, and for an understanding of the unconscious in particular.

The purpose of this volume is to review some of the progress that has been made in the dialogue between those interested in integrating cognitive science and psychodynamic theories and methods. It is not our intention in this book to examine any particular unconscious phenomenon or experimental paradigm in detail; rather, the aim is to present a set of chapters that provide a good representation of work in the field and that offer a flavor of both what has been accomplished and what remains to be done. Our goal was to appeal to both clinicians and researchers.

In the remainder of this chapter, I make some general observations about the intersection of cognitive science and psychoanalysis; these will help introduce and orient succeeding chapters. I note that 1) the dialogue between cognitive science and psychoanalysis, although new, has a long tradition; 2) the dialogue has immediate clinical appeal because both cognitive science and psychoanalysis are multidisciplinary arenas; 3) a number of recent exciting developments—both theoretical (e.g., the implicit/explicit distinction, neural network models of consciousness/unconsciousness) and methodological—have contributed to this dialogue; and 4) a cognitive clinical science may be able to synthesize important philosophical disparities in the way different theorists approach the study of mind.

## Background to the Dialogue

The dialogue between cognitive science and psychoanalysis has been ongoing for some time, albeit in different forms. It may be argued, for example, that there is a strong cognitivist strand in psychoanalysis. Freud himself made a number of significant cognitivist contributions—his conscious-preconscious distinction predates current concepts of accessibility-activation (Erdelyi and Goldberg 1979), he detailed different kinds of cognitive processes (primary versus secondary), and his notion of signal anxiety has a remarkably cybernetic flavor. Although Freud's metapsychology of psychic energetics is clearly not a cognitivist one, a more charitable characterization is that Freud simply lacked the computer metaphor, and that had this metaphor been available to him, there would have been less need for the multiple, often contradictory metaphors of mind that he employed (Erdelyi 1985).

Freud was by no means, however, the first theorist to argue for the existence of an unconscious mind (Ellenberger 1970; Kihlstrom 1987). In particular, the work of Janet has an especially cognitivist flavor (Cloitre, Chapter 3, and Weinberger and Weiss, Chapter 2 in this volume). With remarkable prescience, Janet posited the existence of psychological automatisms—units that combined cognition, emotion, motivation, and action—that were typically accessible to introspection, but that could become dissociated from conscious control. This theoretical framework was revived by Hilgard (1977) and has been expanded by Kihlstrom (1984) to devise a cognitivist approach to dissociative phenomena.

Post-Freudian ego psychologists developed the cognitivist strand in psychoanalysis by contributing to our understanding of ego functions, including cognition (Rapaport 1942). Several psychoanalysts made a particular attempt to emphasize the importance of cognition in psychopathology (Arieti 1965; Barnett 1980; Bieber 1980; Klein 1976; Weiss et al. 1986). Since the work of Sullivan and

Horney, the interpersonal school of psychoanalysis has also emphasized cognitive factors (Crowley 1985; Rendon 1985). The current dominance of object relations psychoanalytic theory might be seen as implicitly cognitivist insofar as it involves an emphasis on self- and other representations (Segal and Blatt 1993).

Since the development of cognitive psychology and artificial intelligence, several psychoanalysts have made explicit attempts to incorporate the constructs and methods of the two fields (Colby and Stoller 1988; Galatzer-Levy 1985; Holt 1964; Palambo 1973; Peterfreund 1971; Pfeifer and Leuzinger-Bohleber 1986; Rosenblatt and Thickstun 1977; Rubinstein 1967; Slap and Slap-Shelton 1991; Teller and Dahl 1985; Westen 1993). Horowitz (1988a, 1988b, 1991, Chapter 8 in this volume) has been particularly influential in encouraging psychoanalysis to forge a link with the constructs and methods of cognitive science.

Conversely, several cognitivists have drawn upon psychodynamic theory. A tradition dating back to Helmholtz (1867/1962) has posited "unconscious inference" in perception, and since Poetzl (1917/1960), a variety of subliminal-stimulus paradigms have been used to investigate unconscious processing (Bruner and Klein 1960; Dixon 1971, 1981; Erdelyi 1974, 1985; Eriksen and Pierce 1968; Holender 1986; Merikle 1982). As mentioned earlier, Hilgard (1977) revived the work of Janet to devise a cognitivist approach to dissociative phenomena. Erdelyi (1985), in an important volume, argued that Freudian theory could be reframed in terms of contemporary cognitive psychology. In the artificial intelligence arena, Wegman (1985) suggested that it would be possible to simulate Freudian theory in a computational model. Indeed, in a remarkable piece of research, Colby (1974) succeeded in developing a computer simulation of the defenses of a paranoid patient.

Investigation of several other topics in cognitive science has also contributed to a bridge with psychoanalysis, albeit less directly. Such areas include work on irrationality (Johnson-Laird 1983; Kahneman and Tversky 1982), automaticity (Hasher and Zacks 1984; LaBerge and Samuels 1974; Posner and Snyder 1975; Shiffrin and Schneider 1977), affect (Oatley and Johnson-Laird 1987; Simon 1967), self-schemas (Markus 1977; Segal and Blatt 1993), and altered states of consciousness such as sleep and hypnosis (Foulkes 1985). Such work confirms the importance of the psycho-dynamic insistence that the human mind cannot be understood as entirely rational or logical, but rather operates in peculiarly biased ways. Gardner (1985) has coined the term "computational para-dox" to refer to the fact that an important lesson of research on the linear-sequential (von Neumann) computational model of the mind is that the human mind works in a more complex way than the model suggests.

Cognitive-behavior therapy does not necessarily draw on cog-nitive science. Nevertheless, certain authors have at times done so explicitly. In addition, a distinction may be made between the first generation of cognitive therapists and a second construc-tivist (Mahoney 1985) or structural (Dobson 1988) generation, which has taken an interest in psychodynamic issues such as transference and affect. This work includes that of Beck et al. (1990), Guidano and Liotto (1983), Joyce-Moniz (1985), A. Ryle (1982), Mahoney (1985), Weiner (1985), Young (1990), and Green-berg and Safran (1987).

A series of recent volumes has further encouraged the dialogue between psychoanalysis and cognitive science (Baars 1992; Bow-ers and Meichenbaum 1984; Bornstein and Pittman 1992; Curtis 1991; Greenwald 1992; Kurtzman, in press; Prigatano and Schach-ter 1991; Segal and Blatt 1993; Singer 1990; Uleman and Bargh 1989). Such works have focused on diverse phenomena—repres-sion and dissociation, slips and errors, and the concept of self—and contemporary research methods for exploring the unconscious.

Despite this long tradition of dialogue, it is important to empha-size that there are significant differences between the so-called cognitive unconscious (Kihlstrom 1987; Rozin 1976; Weiner 1975) and the psychodynamic unconscious. Whereas the psychoanalytic unconscious often refers to a specific psychic structure, the cogni-tive unconscious often refers rather to a type of mental process-ing. The psychoanalytic unconscious is frequently conceptualized as a "boiling pot" of instinctual drives, whereas cognitive uncon-scious processing is typically depicted as structured and automatic (Eagle 1987; Shevrin 1988). The psychoanalytic unconscious is intimately associated with affect and motivation, whereas the cognitive unconscious has broached these constructs only recently. Nevertheless, a dialogue between psychodynamic theory and cognitive science also suggests certain similarities between their approaches (Eagle 1987; Turkle 1988), with both frameworks intent on discovering and detailing the underlying mental structures that produce conscious mental events. Weinberger and Weiss (Chapter 2 in this volume) discuss these contrasts and comparisons in more detail.

## Cognitive Science and Psychoanalysis as Multidisciplinary

Just as a simplistic view of psychoanalysis equates this rich tradition with the work of Freud, so a reductionist view of cognitive science sees that field as concerned only with cognition. The tendency of psychoanalysts to revere Freud, and the term "cognitive science" are perhaps partly responsible for such erroneous characterizations. Nevertheless, both psychoanalysis and cognitive science are much broader than these views would suggest. Indeed, it may be argued that both cognitive science and psychoanalysis are extraordinary academic endeavors in that they self-consciously see themselves as incorporating several scientific disciplines.

Central components of cognitive science include philosophy, cognitive psychology, artificial intelligence, linguistics, neurobiology, anthropology/sociology, and developmental psychology. Cognitive science draws on both the constructs and the methods of these different fields, bringing them together around a focus on computational models of the mind (Gardner 1985; Posner 1989).

Many of the questions currently studied in cognitive science were first raised by philosophy. The continued inclusion of philosophy as a subdiscipline of cognitive science suggests that an additional contribution of philosophy lies in detailing the metatheory of cognitive science itself. Cognitive psychology can be seen as the backbone of cognitive science, providing many of its core theoretical constructs. In particular, cognitive psychology is interested in information processing and representation. Artificial intelligence establishes a rigorous computational methodology for cognitive science—computer simulation. Current work on neural networks in particular has led to an important set of computational models for cognitive science. Cognition and language are intimately related, so that linguistics is an important testing ground for cognitive science research. Neurobiology and anthropology/sociology provide the upper and lower limits, respectively, of the representational level studied in cognitive science.

From the perspective of the clinician, who must deal with each patient at so many different levels, the multidisciplinary nature of cognitive science is an important strength. Similarly, psychoanalytic theory and practice, although based in clinical experience, have from the first incorporated many fields (Kitcher 1992)—with extensive connections to philosophy (Wollheim and Hopkins 1982), linguistics (Lacan 1979), biology (Sulloway 1984), and anthropology (Jahoda 1982). As a multifaceted, complex enterprise, cognitive science has immediate appeal for clinicians and psychoanalytic thinkers interested in new ways of approaching the unconscious.

Several of the authors in this book demonstrate the importance of multidisciplinary thinking. Although the backbone of this book is derived from cognitive psychology (e.g., Cloitre, Chapter 3 in this volume), chapters are included that focus on work from artificial intelligence (e.g., Hoffman, Chapter 5) and linguistics (e.g., Lakoff, Chapter 4 in this volume). Several chapters also emphasize biological findings (e.g., Hoffman, Chapter 5 in this volume). While the problem of integrating diverse fields is clearly not trivial, the attempt to do so is exciting and inspiring.

## Schemas, Neural Networks, and Implicit/Explicit Processing

There are two major models in cognitive science—symbolic and connectionist. The elements of symbolic structures are symbols that are stored in associative structures. Connectionist models, on the other hand, are based on simplified and schematized neurons that are interconnected in a network. Some authors have suggested that only one or the other of these models is valid, with symbolic models, for example, being consistent with a positivist focus on formal laws of information processing while connectionist models allow a more constructivist approach. On the other hand, these two models can be seen as complementary bottom-up and top-down perspectives on the human mind (Dinmore 1992; Rumelhart et al. 1986).

Certainly, at this early point in the history of cognitive science, it would seem prudent to allow for the value of both approaches to the mind. By way of example, both symbolic and connectionist models may be useful in understanding the distinction between implicit and explicit cognitive processing. This distinction is a particularly important one for cognitive science approaches to the unconscious (Cloitre, Chapter 3, and Stein and Young, Chapter 6 in this volume) and deserves a brief introduction here.

Early observations of patients with neurological amnesia indicated that although their ability to recall memories explicitly was impaired, these patients appeared to retain a covert form of the memory. For example, Korsakoff (1889) described an amnesic patient to whom he gave electric shocks during a meeting. Later on, when Korsakoff returned carrying the shock apparatus, the patient—despite retaining no overt memory of either Korsakoff or their earlier meeting—accused Korsakoff of coming to give him electric shocks. Similar examples have been described by Claparède, Janet, Freud, and others (Cloitre, Chapter 3 in this volume). Such examples make it clear that memory involves not only "memory that . . . ," but also "memory how . . . " (cf. Polanyi 1966; G. Ryle 1949). Schachter (1987) has provided a detailed review of how these different kinds of memory have been given a variety of names by different authors, including procedural versus declarative, working versus reference, and semantic versus episodic. The terms implicit and explicit are currently popular.

Kihlstrom (1987) suggested that the implicit/explicit distinction applies not only to memory but also to perception, judgment, learning, and thought. The term *implicit perception*, for example, includes the long-studied phenomenon of subliminal perception. As Poetzl (1917/1960) demonstrated early in this century, stimuli shown for very brief periods with a tachistoscope do not reach consciousness directly but are nevertheless processed. Implicit processing may lead to quite counterintuitive results—as when Pierce and Jastrow (1884) found that subjects' judgments of the relative weight of two similar objects were remarkably accurate despite the fact that they had no explicit awareness of which object was heavier.

Dissociation between implicit and explicit processing has been studied under a variety of circumstances (Kihlstrom 1987). This work leads straightforwardly to a concept of the cognitive unconscious. As Cloitre (Chapter 3 in this volume) suggests, a traumatic experience may be remembered implicitly but not explicitly. As a result, a victim of abuse may deny a particular memory yet manifest symptoms that clearly point to the existence of the memory. Such a phenomenon is reminiscent of Freud's initial work on repression (Stein and Young, Chapter 6 in this volume).

Although the implicit/explicit distinction originates in cognitive psychology, it is readily reframed in the terms of connectionism. Spiegel (1990; Spiegel and Li, Chapter 7 in this volume), for example, has outlined a neural network model of dissociation. In his view, a concept of memories as parallel and distributed—rather than automatically unitary—provides a ready basis for understanding how they can function more or less autonomously. The connectionist view allows an approach to understanding learning as it takes places locally (at the synaptic level) without necessarily requiring the explicit formulation of knowledge (at a more global level).

Indeed, an advantage of neural network models is their ability to incorporate neurobiological knowledge, thereby allowing a type of theorizing that includes both the representational and the neurobiological levels in a seamless way (Hoffman 1987, Chapter 5 in this volume; Park and Young 1994). Conversely, increased understanding of the neurobiology of implicit and explicit processing (Squire 1986) provides impetus for the development of connectionist models of their dissociation.

# Methodological Advances

Despite theoretical advances in cognitive approaches to unconscious processing, the skeptic may raise the thorny question of measurement. The clinical data provided by so many as a basis for the hypothesis of an unconscious have been derided as unreliable and unreplicable. On the other hand, laboratory studies using meaningless stimuli (e.g., Ebbinghaus's [1885] nonsense words) do not seem to provide the complexity required for a clinically relevant science of the unconscious.

Cognitive science is, however, becomingly increasingly adept at using different kinds of methodologies for inferring unconscious processes. Stimuli are now, in the tradition of Bartlett's (1932) studies of memory, meaningful and complex. Methodologies are not limited to the collection of cognitive data but include physiological measures (Shevrin 1988). There is increasing emphasis on individual differences in unconscious processing (Singer 1990).

Nevertheless, for experimental findings to have clinical relevance, explicit attention must be accorded to psychopathology. Attempts are increasingly being made to focus on cognitive processing of affective and conflictual material (Bornstein and Pittman 1992). Although further integration is required, such research has helped to close the gap between the experimentalist and the clinician.

Most recently, there has been an important effort to apply cognitive science concepts and methods within the clinical setting. Horowitz (1988b, Chapter 8 in this volume) has pioneered such work. This research requires significant adaptation of laboratory paradigms, with the development of novel rating scales and systems. Horowitz (1988b) has discussed a method of combining multiple data sets, including cognitive and physiological parameters, to measure inferred unconscious processes. Although labor intensive, this research seems to have significant promise.

# Synthesis of Positivism and Hermeneutics

Psychoanalysis entails a perennial ambivalence for theorists. There is, on the one hand, a temptation to approach psychoanalysis by way of the positivist principles formulated for the investigation of physical systems and the explanation of mechanisms. On the other hand, the hermeneutic principles that apply to the interpretation of literary texts and to the understanding of meanings also seem suitable (Ricoeur 1970). Thus, the positivist might argue that the operations of the unconscious can be rigorously defined, that these mechanisms obey formal laws, and that the unconscious is ultimately explicable in terms of its psychophysical substrate. Conversely, the hermeneuticist may argue that the narrative produced by the unconscious invariably has numerous meanings, that this text requires interpretive understanding rather than simply explanation, and that the study of the unconscious is a human science that cannot be reduced to a natural science.

Clearly, this heuristic polarization of the positivist and hermeneutic positions is an oversimplified division that is most likely unable to capture the work of any particular theorist. Nevertheless, debate between positivist and hermeneutic viewpoints is an important theme running through the social sciences (Keat and Urry 1982). Within psychology, behaviorism can be seen as adopting the fundamental tenets of positivism—a concern with defining meaning in terms of verification (operational definition), with describing the laws that account for various phenomena, and with reducing high-level abstract concepts to basic physical ones. On the other hand, there is a hermeneutic trend in psychology that argues that mental processes are always constructive, that human behavior requires understanding rather than explanation, and that such understanding has more similarities to textual analysis than to scientific experiment (Manicas and Secord 1983).

Cognitive science also faces appropriation by either positivist or hermeneutic principles (Lyddon 1992; Stein 1992b). A purely positivist cognitive science will be interested primarily in symbol manipulation, will attempt to deduce the laws of such transformation, and may argue that the level of information processing is a "basic" level. In contrast, there is also a constructivist movement in cognitive science that emphasizes that cognition cannot be limited to symbol manipulation, focuses on the interactive context rather than simply on symbol transformation, and argues that it is important to consider not only the level of information representation but also the levels of physical substrate and social context (Neisser 1976; Norman 1993).

These positions are idealizations that do, however, point to the importance of an integrative approach to the unconscious. A positivist approach to the unconscious, whether based on psychic energetics or on symbol transformation, runs the risk of missing the importance of meaning in the human mind, of social context, and of the complex interaction between biological and psychological levels. A hermeneutic approach to the unconscious, whether based on psychoanalytic constructs or on cognitive constructivism, runs the risk of relegating unconscious mechanisms to mere narrative devices.

An integrative or synthetic approach seems difficult. Nevertheless, I would suggest that insofar as cognitive science is successful in providing powerful explanations of the mind and the unconscious, it will concomitantly synthesize the best aspects of both positivism and hermeneutics. Good natural science necessarily involves understanding real mechanisms in the world; good social science also deals with human meanings and contexts.

Several authors in this volume provide just such an integrative approach to the unconscious. Lakoff (1987, Chapter 4 in this volume), for example, is able to describe the grammar of the unconscious in terms that address both mechanism and meaning. He has taken pains to contrast his approach with positivist approaches that view mental operations as algorithmic. Lakoff (1987) has made a fundamental contribution to cognitive science by arguing that language, and categorization in particular, cannot be understood by means of algorithmic approaches based on positivist principles. Instead, Lakoff emphasizes the importance of metaphor in understanding language and categorization—metaphor that does not simply entail straightforward transformative laws but that rather reflects human experience, pointing to the embodiment of mind in the brain and in social context. Nevertheless, although Lakoff is intimately concerned with meaning and interaction, he sees himself as a scientist who is trying to understand the mechanisms of the mind rather than as a literary critic. His work thus synthesizes—in the same way that good clinical theory and practice do—both mechanism and meaning.

The theme of clinical science drawing on the concepts and methods of cognitive science runs throughout much of this volume. However, it is important not to neglect what the clinic offers cognitivists. Too often, textbooks of cognitive science make little or no reference to psychopathology. It is an obvious point that theories of mind are incomplete if they cannot also explain aberrations of the mind. Even more important, however, is the notion that an adequate understanding of psychopathology demands a complex, integrative approach to the mind. The synthesis of mechanism and meaning by Lakoff and others in this volume represents an important goal for cognitive science as a whole.

## Conclusion

I have indicated that the dialogue between cognitive science and psychoanalysis has a long tradition and continues to develop in several ways. The chapters of this book illustrate these advances and point to the ways in which further progress is likely to occur. Important theoretical advances have been made in this dialogue, and new methodological developments allow empirical testing of these theories.

I would argue that a reframing of psychoanalytic concepts in terms of the multidisciplinary constructs of cognitive science allows us to go beyond an outdated metapsychology. (For an alternative view, however, see the work of Weinberger and Weiss, Chapter 2 in this volume). Conversely, retaining psychoanalytic complexity in our cognitive research allows us to go beyond sterile laboratory paradigms. Taken together, work in cognitive science and psychoanalysis can lead to an integrative, synthetic approach that incorporates the best of the positivist and hermeneutic views of the mind.

Several areas require further investigation. While this volume focuses on areas of clinical relevance, further work is needed on the application of this knowledge to clinical assessment and evaluation (Horowitz, Chapter 8 in this volume). An understanding of the unconscious also requires improved knowledge of consciousness (Hoffman, Chapter 5 in this volume; Marcel 1983). Empirical investigation of the cognitive unconscious is still at an early stage—much additional work remains to be done (Weinberger and Weiss, Chapter 2 in this volume). This volume reflects current progress; we look forward to further advances in the dialogue between cognitive science and the unconscious.

# References

Arieti S: Contributions to cognition from psychoanalytic theory, in Science and Psychoanalysis, Vol 3. Edited by Masserman J. New York, Grune & Stratton, 1965

Baars BJ: The Cognitive Revolution in Psychology. New York, Guilford, 1986

Baars BJ (ed): Experimental Slips and Human Error: Exploring the Architecture of Volition. New York, Plenum, 1992

Barnett J: Cognitive repair in the treatment of neurosis. J Am Acad Psychoanal 8:39–56, 1980

Bartlett FC: Remembering: A Study in Experimental and Social Psychology. Cambridge, UK, Cambridge University Press, 1932

Beck AT, Freeman A, Pretzer J, et al: Cognitive Therapy of Personality Disorders. New York, Guilford, 1990

Bhaskar R: A Realist Theory of Science, 2nd Edition. Sussex, UK, Harvester Press, 1978

Bieber I: Psychoanalysis—a cognitive process. J Am Acad Psychoanal 8:25–38, 1980

Bornstein RF, Pittman TS (eds): Perception Without Awareness: Cognitive, Clinical, and Social Perspectives. New York, Guilford, 1992

Bowers KS, Meichenbaum D (eds): The Unconscious Reconsidered. New York, Wiley, 1984

Bruner JS, Klein GS: The function of perceiving: New Look retrospect, in Perspectives in Psychological Theory. Edited by Wapner S, Kaplan B. New York, International Universities Press, 1960, pp 61–77

Colby KM: Artificial Paranoia. New York, Pergamon, 1974

Colby KM, Stoller RJ: Cognitive Science and Psychoanalysis. Hillsdale, NJ, Analytic Press, 1988

Crowley RM: Cognition in interpersonal theory and practice, in Cognition and Psychotherapy. Edited by Mahoney MJ, Freeman A. New York, Plenum, 1985, pp 291–312

Curtis RC (ed): The Relational Self: Theoretical Convergences of Psychoanalysis and Social Psychology. New York, Guilford, 1991

Dinmore J (ed): The Symbolic and Connectionist Paradigms. Hillsdale, NJ, Lawrence Erlbaum, 1992

Dixon NF: Subliminal Processing: The Nature of a Controversy. New York, McGraw-Hill, 1971

Dixon NF: Preconscious Processing. New York, Wiley, 1981

Dobson KS (ed): Handbook of Cognitive-Behavioral Therapies. New York, Guilford, 1988

Dollard J, Miller N: Personality and Psychotherapy. New York, McGraw-Hill, 1950

Eagle MN: The psychoanalytic and the cognitive unconscious, in Theories of the Unconscious and Theories of the Self. Edited by Stern R. Hillsdale, NJ, Lawrence Erlbaum, 1987, pp 155–190

Ebbinghaus H: Memory. Translated by Ruger HA, Bussenius CE. New York, Dover, 1964 (original work published in 1885)

Ellenberger HF: The Rediscovery of the Unconscious: The History and Evolution of Dynamic Psychiatry. New York, Basic Books, 1970

Erdelyi MH: A new look at the New Look: perceptual defense and vigilance. Psychol Rev 81:1–25, 1974

Erdelyi MH: Psychoanalysis: Freud's Cognitive Psychology. New York, WH Freeman, 1985

Erdelyi MH, Goldberg B: Let's not sweep repression under the rug: toward a cognitive psychology of repression, in Functional Disorders of Memory. Edited by Kihlstrom JF, Evans FJ. Hillsdale, NJ, Lawrence Erlbaum, 1979, pp 355–402

Eriksen C, Pierce J: Defense mechanisms, in Handbook of Personality Theory and Research. Edited by Borgatta E, Lambert W. Chicago, IL, Rand McNally, 1968

Foulkes D: Dreaming: A Cognitive-Psychological Analysis. Hillsdale, NJ, Lawrence Erlbaum, 1985

Freud S: Some elementary lessons in psychoanalysis (1938), in General Psychological Theory: Papers on Metapsychology. New York, Collier Books, 1963

Galatzer-Levy RM: On working through: a model from artificial intelligence. J Am Psychoanal Assoc 33:125–151, 1985

Gardner H: The Mind's New Science: A History of the Cognitive Revolution. New York, Basic Books, 1985

Greenberg LS, Safran JD: Emotion in Psychotherapy. New York, Guilford, 1987

Greenwald AG: New look 3: unconscious cognition reclaimed. Am Psychol 47:766–779, 1992

Grunbaum A: Validation in the Clinical Theory of Psychoanalysis. New York, International Universities Press, 1993

Guidano VF, Liotti G: Cognitive Processes and Emotional Disorders: A Structural Approach to Psychotherapy. New York, Guilford, 1983

Hasher L, Zacks RT: Automatic and effortful processes in memory. J Exp Psychol Gen 108:356–388, 1984

Helmholtz H: Treatise on Physiological Optics, Vol 3 (1867). New York, Dover, 1962

Hilgard ER: Divided Consciousness: Multiple Controls in Human Thought and Action. New York, Wiley, 1977

Hoffman RE: Computer simulations of neural information processing and the schizophrenia–mania dichotomy. Arch Gen Psychiatry 44:178–188, 1987

Holender D: Semantic activation without conscious identification in dichotic listening, parafoveal vision, and visual masking: a survey and appraisal. Behavioral and Brain Sciences 9:1–66, 1986

Holt R: The emergence of cognitive psychology. J Am Psychoanal Assoc 12:650–665, 1964

Horowitz MJ: Introduction to Psychodynamics: A New Synthesis. New York, Basic Books, 1988a

Horowitz MJ (ed): Psychodynamics and Cognition. Chicago, IL, University of Chicago Press, 1988b

Horowitz MJ (ed): Person Schemas and Maladaptive Interpersonal Patterns. Chicago, IL, University of Chicago Press, 1991

Jahoda G: Psychology and Anthropology: A Psychological Perspective. New York, Academic Press, 1982

Johnson-Laird PN: Mental Models: Towards a Cognitive Science of Language, Inference, and Consciousness. Cambridge, MA, Harvard University Press, 1983

Joyce-Moniz L: Epistemological therapy and constructivism, in Cognition and Psychotherapy. Edited by Mahoney MJ, Freeman A. New York, Plenum, 1985, pp 143–180

Kahneman D, Tversky A: The psychology of preferences. Sci Am 246:160–174, 1982

Keat R, Urry J: Social Theory as Science, 2nd Edition. London, Routledge & Kegan Paul, 1982

Kihlstrom JF: Conscious, subconscious, unconscious: a cognitive perspective, in The Unconscious Reconsidered. Edited by Bowers KS, Meichenbaum D. New York, Wiley, 1984, pp 149–211

Kihlstrom JF: The cognitive unconscious. Science 237:1445–1452, 1987

Kitcher P: Freud's Dream: A Complete Interdisciplinary Science of Mind. New York, Bradford, 1992

Klein GS: Psychoanalytic Theory: An Exploration of Essentials. New York, International Universities Press, 1976

Korsakoff SS: Etude medico-psychologique sur une forme des maladies de la memoire. Revue Philosophique 28:501–530, 1889

Kurtzman H (ed): Cognition and Psychodynamics: New Perspectives. New York, Oxford University Press (in press)

LaBerge D, Samuels SJ: Toward a theory of automatic information processing in reading. Cognitive Psychology 6:293–323, 1974

Lacan J: The Four Fundamental Concepts of Psychoanalysis. Harmondsworth, Middlesex, UK, Penguin, 1979

Lakoff G: Women, Fire, and Dangerous Things: What Categories Reveal About the Mind. Chicago, IL, University of Chicago Press, 1987

Lyddon WJ: Cognitive science and psychotherapy: an epistemic framework, in Cognitive Science and Clinical Disorders. Edited by Stein DJ, Young JE. San Diego, CA, Academic Press, 1992, pp 173–187

Mahoney MJ: Psychotherapy and human change processes, in Cognition and Psychotherapy. Edited by Mahoney MJ, Freeman A. New York, Plenum, 1985, pp 3–48

Manicas PT, Secord PF: Implications for psychology of the new philosophy of science. Am Psychol 33:399–413, 1983

Marcel AJ: Conscious and unconscious perception: an approach to the relations between phenomenal experience and perceptual processes. Cognitive Psychology 15:238–300, 1983

Markus H: Self-schemata and processing information about the self. J Pers Soc Psychol 35:63–78, 1977

Merikle PM: Unconscious perception revisited. Perception and Psychophysics 31:298–301, 1982

Neisser U: Cognition and Reality: Principles and Implications of Cognitive Science. San Francisco, CA, WH Freeman, 1976

Norman DA: Cognition in the head and in the world: an introduction to the special issue on situated action. Cognition 17:1–6, 1993

Oatley K, Johnson-Laird PN: Towards a cognitive theory of emotion. Cognition and Emotion 1:29–50, 1987

Palambo S: The associative memory tree, in Psychoanalysis and Contemporary Science, Vol 2. Edited by Rubinstein BB. New York, Macmillan, 1973

Park SBG, Young AH: Connectionism and psychiatry: a brief review. Philosophy, Psychiatry, and Psychology 1:51–58, 1994

Peterfreund E: Information, Systems, and Psychoanalysis: An Evolutionary Biological Approach to Psychoanalytic Theory. New York, International Universities Press, 1971

Pfeifer R, Leuzinger-Bohleber M: Applications of cognitive science methods to psychoanalysis: a case study and some theory. Int Rev Psychoanal 13:221–240, 1986

Pierce CS, Jastrow J: On small differences in sensation. Memoirs of the National Academy of Science 3:75–83, 1884

Poetzl O: The relationship between experimentally induced dream images and indirect vision (1917), in Preconscious Stimulation in Dreams, Associations, and Images: Classical Studies (Psychological Issues 2, monograph 7). Edited by Fisher C. New York, International Universities Press, 1960, pp 46–106

Polanyi M: The Tacit Dimension. Garden City, NY, Doubleday, 1966

Posner MI (ed): The Foundations of Cognitive Science. Cambridge, MA, MIT Press, 1989

Posner MI, Snyder CRR: Attention and cognitive control, in Information Processing in Cognition: The Loyola Symposium. Edited by Solso RL. Hillsdale, NJ, Lawrence Erlbaum, 1975, pp 55–85

Prigatano GP, Schachter DL (eds): Awareness of Deficit After Brain Injury: Clinical and Theoretical Issues. New York, Oxford University Press, 1991

Rapaport D: Emotions and Memory. New York, International Universities Press, 1942

Rendon M: Cognition and psychoanalysis: a Horneyean perspective, in Cognition and Psychotherapy. Edited by Mahoney MJ, Freeman A. New York, Plenum, 1985, pp 277–290

Ricoeur P: Freud and Philosophy: An Essay on Interpretation. New Haven, CT, Yale University Press, 1970

Rosenblatt AD, Thickstun JT: Energy, information, and motivation: a revision of psychoanalytic theory. J Am Psychoanal Assoc 25:529–558, 1977

Rozin P: The evolution of intelligence and access to the cognitive unconscious. Progress in Psychobiology and Physiological Psychology 6:245–280, 1976

Rubinstein BB: Explanation and mere description: a metascientific examination of certain aspects of the psychoanalytic theory of motivation, in Motives and Thought (Psychological Issues, monograph 18/19). Edited by Holt RR. New York, International Universities Press, 1967

Rumelhart DE, Smolensky P, McClelland JL, et al: Schemata and sequential thought processes in PDP models, in Parallel Distributed Processing: Explorations in the Microstructure of Cognition, Vol 2: Physiological and Biological Models. Edited by McClelland JL, Rumelhart DE, PDP Research Group. Cambridge, MA, MIT Press, 1986, pp 7–57

Ryle A: Psychotherapy: A Cognitive Integration of Theory and Practise. London, Academic Press, 1982

Ryle G: The Concept of Mind. London, Hutchinson, 1949

Schachter DL: Implicit memory: history and current status. J Exp Psychol Learn Mem Cogn 13:501–518, 1987

Segal ZV, Blatt SJ (eds): The Self in Emotional Distress: Cognitive and Psychodynamic Perspectives. New York, Guilford, 1993

Shevrin H: Unconscious conflict: a convergent psychodynamic and electrophysiological approach, in Psychodynamics and Cognition. Edited by Horowitz MJ. Chicago, IL, University of Chicago Press, 1988, pp 117–168

Shiffrin RM, Schneider W: Controlled and automatic human information processing, II: perceptual learning, automatic attending, and a general theory. Psychol Rev 84:127–190, 1977

Simon H: Motivational and emotional controls of cognition. Psychol Rev 74:29–39, 1967

Singer JL (ed): Repression and Dissociation: Implications for Personality Theory, Psychopathology, and Health. Chicago, IL, University of Chicago Press, 1990

Slap JW, Slap-Shelton L: The Schema in Clinical Psychoanalysis. Hillsdale, NJ, Analytic Press, 1991

Spiegel D: Hypnosis, dissociation, and trauma: hidden and overt observers, in Repression and Dissociation: Implications for Personality Theory, Psychopathology, and Health. Edited by Singer JL. Chicago, IL, University of Chicago Press, 1990, pp 121–142

Squire LR: Mechanisms of memory. Science 232:1612–1619, 1986

Stein DJ: Psychoanalysis and cognitive science: contrasting models of the mind. J Am Acad Psychoanal 20:543–559, 1992a

Stein DJ: Cognitive science and clinical knowledge. Integrative Psychiatry 8:109–116, 1992b

Stein DJ: Cognitive science and psychiatry: an overview. Integrative Psychiatry 9:13–24, 1994

Sulloway F: Freud, Biologist of the Mind. New York, Basic Books, 1984

Teller V, Dahl H: The microstructure of free association. J Am Acad Psychoanal 33:763–798, 1985

Turkle S: Artificial intelligence and psychoanalysis: a new alliance. Daedalus 1988, pp 241–268

Uleman JS, Bargh JA (eds): Unintended Thought. New York, Guilford, 1989

Wegman C: Psychoanalysis and Cognitive Psychology: A Formalization of Freud's Earliest Theory. London, Academic Press, 1985

Weiner ML: The Cognitive Unconscious: A Piagetian Approach to Psychotherapy. Davis, CA, International Psychological Press, 1975

Weiner ML: Cognitive-Experiential Therapy: An Integrative Ego Psychotherapy. New York, Brunner/Mazel, 1985

Weiss J, Sampson H, Mount Zion Psychotherapy Research Group: The Psychoanalytic Process: Theory, Clinical Observation, and Empirical Research. New York, Guilford, 1986

Westen D: Transference and information processing, in Essential Papers in Transference Analysis. Edited by Bauer G. Northvale, NJ, Jason Aronson, 1993, pp 19–51

Widiger TA: Book review: *Borderline Personality Disorder: Etiology and Treatment* (Edited by Paris J. Washington, DC, American Psychiatric Press, 1992). Am J Psychiatry 151:1244, 1994

Wollheim R, Hopkins J: Philosophical Essays on Freud. Cambridge, UK, Cambridge University Press, 1982

Young JE: Cognitive Therapy for Personality Disorders: A Schema-Focused Approach. Sarasota, FL, Professional Resource Exchange, 1990

# Chapter 2

# *Psychoanalytic and Cognitive Conceptions of the Unconscious*

Joel Weinberger, Ph.D., and Joshua Weiss, Ph.D.

Mental health professionals have long made use of models of the mind that viewed unconscious processes as central to human functioning. The major clinical model used in this way has historically been psychoanalysis. In contrast, academic psychologists have traditionally not studied unconscious processes, often denying their existence altogether (Weinberger, in preparation). With the demise of behaviorism and the rise of the so-called cognitive revolution, unconscious processes are once again in fashion in the academic community. But the unconscious being propounded in these circles differs from psychoanalytic notions of the unconscious. This creates a dilemma for the clinician. Which model should be used? Which model is correct? Which model offers the better way to understand our patients?

In this chapter, we review psychoanalytic and cognitive conceptions of unconscious processes. We point out where they converge and, perhaps more importantly, where they diverge. We then briefly discuss some recent efforts to integrate the two. Finally, we offer our conclusions as to the place of each of these models in understanding the human mind and in treating our patients.

Because this chapter is largely a theoretical one, we focus our attention on the theoretical writings of the various proponents of the cognitive and psychoanalytic points of view. We also exam-

Preparation of this chapter was supported in part by National Institute of Mental Health First Award Grant 1 R29 MH48955-01A1 to Dr. Weinberger.

ine empirical research when we believe it may shed light on these theoretical issues.

# Psychoanalytic Conceptions of the Unconscious

No single psychoanalytic conception of the unconscious exists, just as no single psychoanalytic theory exists. As nearly as we can determine, there are four major views on unconscious processing in this tradition. Two come from classical psychoanalysis and have been termed the *topographical* and the *structural* models. The other two stem from object relations theory and self psychology, respectively.

## Classical Psychoanalysis: The Topographical Model

The topographical model proposes a tripartite division of the mind into conscious, preconscious, and unconscious systems. It is most clearly laid out in Chapter 7 of Freud's "Interpretation of Dreams" and a metapsychological paper written years later (Freud 1900/ 1953, 1915/1957). The basis of the division concerns the availability of mental contents to awareness.

The conscious system contains all that a person is aware of at any time. Information potentially available to but not currently held in awareness resides in a preconscious system. The rules of operation of these two systems are similar, and so the flow of information from one to the other is relatively free and effortless. As a result, Freud sometimes referred to the conscious system and the preconscious system as a single preconscious-conscious system.

The unconscious system is another story. Its operation is qualitatively different from that of the preconscious-conscious system(s), and none of its contents are available to awareness. At its core are inborn drives or instincts, most prominently the sexual drive (an aggressive drive was later added [Freud 1920/1955]). These drives continually press for expression, manifested as wishes or desires needing to be met. Such desires are not affected by practical considerations. Nor does the fact that satisfying some desires would thwart others affect their constant efforts to be met. They all strive simultaneously for fulfillment, heedless of possible consequences.

They are also relatively unaffected by developmental changes, the passage of time, or changes in circumstance. Night, day, asleep, awake, infant, aged—it makes no difference. This system consists only of desires pressing to be fulfilled, and they are relentless.

The purpose of all this striving is to discharge drive tension, which is experienced as painful. The discharge of such tension is pleasurable, and the unconscious system will agree to anything that will foster this discharge. This statement summarizes the pleasure principle. In the service of this principle, one means of discharge may be replaced by another—a phenomenon termed *displacement*. If a means is found that will allow for expression of more than one desire, so much the better. Such a mechanism is termed *condensation*.

Two incompatible wishes may combine to be expressed in a manner intermediate between the two, a sort of compromise between them. This flow of desires through myriad means of expression is termed *primary process* and represents the basic law of the unconscious system and therefore of unconscious processing.

Because environmental stimulation has relatively clear access to the unconscious system, the effects of external reality can be used to fulfill unconscious wishes in line with the pleasure principle. The drives thus become connected with—and the person comes to unconsciously value—whatever in the environment facilitates expression of his or her unconscious wishes. For example, a mother, by virtue of satisfying many of her infant's needs, becomes highly valued and the object of many of its desires. In this way, many unconscious wishes come to revolve around actual people and objects in the real world.

In the real world, environmental and social constraints prevent the free expression of drives, and the desires of the unconscious system are often thwarted. Indeed, satisfying such desires could lead to dangerous consequences—for example, a mother cannot unfailingly meet every desire of her infant, and an adult who attempts to satisfy sexual urges on his mother or an unwilling other will soon be in serious trouble. The preconscious-conscious systems protect the organism from him- or herself and try to arrange for desires to be satisfied in an adaptive manner. They do this by monitoring unconscious desires and attempting to control or censor their access to consciousness. Efforts are made to delay meeting desires that are impractical at the moment and to prohibit those whose expression could have negative consequences. This regulatory function is called *secondary process*. The wishes that do not pass muster are thrust back into the unconscious system. Freud termed this phenomenon *repression*. Because the conscious system controls motor activity, the person cannot act on his or her desires unless and until those desires enter the conscious system. Even the desires that do become represented in the conscious system are usually pale copies of the original wishes. They are disguised, distorted, and/or compromised in some fashion by the guardian censor. These watered-down conscious representations are termed *derivatives* or *substitute formations* to reflect their distorted natures.

Repression is often not completely effective and can be partly overcome. This partial overcoming of repression occurs regularly in jokes, parapraxes, and dreams. In the cases of jokes and parapraxes, a disguised version of a wish is briefly expressed and just as briefly renounced. This disguised expression represents a harmless blowing off of psychic steam, so to speak. In dreams, the censor determines that expression and satisfaction of a wish would be relatively harmless because the satisfaction is private and hallucinatory.

Partial failure of repression can be manifested in one other way—in the formation of symptoms. Symptom formation is not harmless; the person suffers for it. What happens is that the censor weakens and/or the unconscious wish so grows in power that its derivative literally forces its way past an overmatched censor, which nonetheless attempts to stop the wish as best it can. The conflict between the wish and the censor often leads to further distortion and thus to a singularly unsatisfying expression of the underlying wish. This unsatisfactory compromise often results in the symptom that brings the patient into treatment.

This understanding of the mind led to a way of alleviating the suffering of the patient. If the unconscious wish could be made available to awareness, there would be no need for repression, and the symptom would become unnecessary. The risk that the person would act on the wish in dangerous ways is not a serious concern because virtually all repression originates in early childhood, when the psychic apparatus is weak and the child is relatively helpless and dependent. As the child matures, he or she becomes more and more capable of fulfilling desires in an adaptive manner, and so represses less. The adult has even greater and more varied resources, enabling him or her to find more adaptive ways of dealing with wishes. As a result, making an unconscious wish conscious is unlikely to result in negative consequences. More likely, doing so will free up resources and allow the person to function more adaptively and happily.

The method Freud created to achieve these aims was termed *psychoanalysis*. He developed the techniques of free association and dream analysis to allow patients to verbalize and thereby make conscious their unconscious derivatives. Free association involves having the patient relax (lie on a couch with the analyst out of sight) and report anything and everything that comes to mind, regardless of whatever resistance she or he may feel to doing so. Analysis of dreams involves reporting a dream and free-associating to its elements. The analyst is neutral, nonjudgmental, and noninterfering throughout this process. Such an atmosphere fosters feelings of safety and relaxation. The injunction to speak without holding back is designed to overcome the objections of the now relatively relaxed and secure preconscious-conscious censor. Of course, the censor does not cease its activity altogether. The analyst must therefore ask clarifying questions and offer interpretations designed to overcome these the censor's resistances. She or he must also be on the lookout for parapraxes and nonverbal behaviors that might betray the patient's true unconscious intent.

Once repression has been abrogated in this way, unconscious derivatives will enter the conscious system. Distortion and compromise then become less necessary. The actual instigating wish may even achieve consciousness. The symptom will then have no purpose and will cease to exist. The goal of psychoanalysis in the topographical model is therefore to make the unconscious conscious.

## Classical Psychoanalysis: The Structural Model

The topographical model is conceptually tight and easy to follow. Mental content can be characterized by its level of consciousness. Those elements not available to awareness are unconscious by definition and consist of wishes seeking expression. Anything unconscious must be a wish and as such must follow the rules of primary process in the service of the pleasure principle. The clinical task is to make the unconscious conscious.

Unfortunately, this neat formulation did not fit the clinical facts as Freud later saw them. This problem was presaged in Freud's 1915 paper and received full-blown treatment in his structural model of the mind, introduced in its complete form in 1923.

What caused Freud to alter his position was his realization that the operation of the censor in his topographical model was unconscious. Given that he had placed the censor in the preconscious system, it should have been readily available to awareness. But it was not. Serious analytic work was required to make it conscious. The censor resisted being made conscious, and its resistances were also unconscious. This discrepancy could not be resolved by the simple expedient of declaring the censor to be part of the unconscious system, because it did not consist of libidinal and (since 1920) aggressive wishes. Furthermore, Freud found that many moral injunctions set up against the person's desires were also unconscious. These, too, were supposed to be part of the preconscious system and could not be made to fit into the unconscious system of the topographical model.

Freud (1923/1961) solved these problems with an entirely new conception of the mind. Level of consciousness was no longer the key; function became predominant. This conceptualization was termed the structural model, although it could perhaps more accurately be termed the functional model.

In the new structural model, what had been called the unconscious system became the id. It contained the drives, was governed by primary process, and was almost entirely unconscious. This represented little more than a change in terminology. Real changes were evident in what had once been the preconscious-conscious system(s), however. This became the ego, postulated to contain both material generally unavailable and material available to awareness. The methods by which id impulses are dealt with are unconscious. These impulses are termed *defenses* and are at the border of the id and ego, much as the censor was at the border of the unconscious and preconscious-conscious systems. Now however, as a result of their unconscious state, they, too, must be brought into awareness through clinical work. Before the clinician can access an unconscious wish, she or he must make the resistances and defenses used to distort and withhold the wish from consciousness available to awareness. As components of the ego, resistances and defenses are not aspects of wishes but reactions to them. They do not exhibit all of the attributes of primary process, nor are they entirely at the service of the pleasure principle. Defenses possess some primary-process characteristics in that they function, in part, to allay anxiety (Freud 1926/1959), thereby following the pleasure principle. But they also show some secondary-process characteristics in that they have a relation in time and to reality. Resistances and defenses thus fall somewhere between primary and secondary process.

Freud found that moral thinking also had a strong unconscious component. Freud termed the moral aspect of the mind the superego. Although the superego was conceptualized as part of the ego, its operation more strongly resembles id than ego functioning—that is, it is irrational and cares little for reality considerations. Its demands are often unreasonable. Its power derives from aggressive impulses. A patient's moral convictions are often set in direct opposition to id wishes, and little quarter is given by either. As both id and superego demands are unremitting, it is the ego's job to mediate between them.

The structural model is messier than—not as conceptually tight as—the topographical model. Unconscious processes exist in all agencies of the mind. There is no strict set of rules for all unconscious dynamics. Instead, unconscious processes exist on a continuum from primary to secondary process. The structural model is more clinically relevant than the topographical model, however, in that it attempts to address the actual issues and phenomena exhibited by patients and seen by therapists. (Space limits further discussion of the relative merits of the two models here. See Arlow and Brenner 1964 for an excellent comparison of them.) Clinically, the task has changed from an exclusive focus on making the unconscious conscious to the more varied goal of bringing resistances, defenses, and superego injunctions under greater ego control. This must occur before unconscious wishes can be dealt with. Freud therefore said that where id was, there ego shall be. In terms of technique, an increased focus on interpretation over passively attending to free association would be warranted. Such modifications are apparent in the work of Reich (1933/1976) and Brenner (1982). (Also see Arlow and Brenner 1964 for an extended discussion of these treatment implications.)

The structural model has remained relatively unchanged by more modern classical psychoanalysts. The ego psychologists (e.g., Rapaport 1960) extended the power of the ego but otherwise left the structural model intact. Brenner (1982), a prominent classical psychoanalyst, eliminated instincts and tension reduction from the model and replaced them with wishes and their expression. The rest of the model remains untouched and continues to be a viable model for classical psychoanalysts.

## Object Relations Theory

Object relations theory contains too many disparate viewpoints to allow discussion of a single object relational conception of the unconscious. (Greenberg and Mitchell [1983] have reviewed many of the models.) Here we focus on Kernberg's (1976, 1981, 1987) version because we believe that it offers the clearest object relational perspective of unconscious processes. It is also arguably the most influential object relations point of view extant today.

Kernberg begins with two major points to build his theory of object relations. The first has been attributed to Fairbairn (1952) and has become almost axiomatic to object relational conceptions. This point states that there are no drives without objects—that is, wishes have to be about something or directed toward something. And this something is almost always some important relational figure. For Kernberg, this means that the id is composed not of warded-off drives but of repressed representations of drive-infused relationships. (Kernberg calls these representations *repressed internalized object relations.*) It also means that the id is more organized than is implied by classical psychoanalysis and its conception of primary process. Activity cannot be as diffuse and amorphous as the classicists believe if wishes come complete with objects and if desires contain the means of their satisfaction. Condensation and displacement would then not be as free.

The second major point of object relations theory comes from Freud's (1924/1961) observation that the deepest, most repressed id material sometimes reaches consciousness in nonpsychotic patients. This finding led Freud (1940/1964) to postulate a process whereby the structural integrity of the ego could be compromised. This process was termed "splitting" and suggests that the ego and id are not as strongly differentiated as Freud originally thought. Kernberg (1975) made the phenomenon of splitting central to his understanding and treatment of borderline pathology. Although delineation of the splitting process probably constitutes his greatest contribution to clinical work, splitting is not vital to our discussion of the unconscious, and we therefore will not pursue it further here. For our purposes, the important point is that id and ego can be relatively undifferentiated from one another and are not as qualitatively different as the classicists believe. This point is reinforced by the axiomatic object relations belief previously described (i.e., that all desires pertain to relationships).

According to Kernberg, mental life begins with inborn propensities to relate and to form representations of relationships. The form these propensities take depends on the interaction of the person's actual relational experiences and his or her maturing cognitive capabilities. At first, affectively powerful experiences are most salient. The developing infant therefore structures experience around gratifications and frustrations. Because this organization is affectively based, parallel organizations can develop around the same object. One configuration is based on positive experiences, the other on negative experiences. Because the mother is the source of most important early interactions, these early schemas focus on her. Thus, the infant develops a conception of the "good" mother in parallel to one of the "bad" mother. The infant is not aware that the object of these feelings is the same person; it is aware only of powerful feelings that are diametrically opposed to one another. Even this awareness is only rudimentary. The infant knows that it has feelings, but it is not self-aware—that is, there is not yet an "I" who has these feelings. Kernberg refers to this primitive state of awareness as a *rudimentary id–ego matrix* because the two structures are totally undifferentiated at this point.

As positive and negative affective experiences accumulate, each set begins to become more completely organized and structured. Gratifying, positive experiences, which are largely sensual and sexual, cohere into what classicists would term *libido,* or the sexual drive. Frustrating, negative experiences, which are largely aggressive, cohere into the aggressive drive. Thus, in Kernberg's model, affect and relationships precede the development of drives. In the classical model, the sequence is exactly the opposite: first are the drives or wishes, which then attach themselves to objects through the primary process.

The mind gradually becomes more organized. The next step is for less-charged relational experiences to become represented. This process is a function of the increasing number of opportunities for interaction and the infant's maturing cognitive capabilities. As such enhanced representation develops, the infant can begin to recognize that some of its all-good and all-bad representations refer to the same person. There is also greater recognition of what differentiates the self from others, thereby allowing for some integration of these representations. A rudimentary sense of self (an "I") and of others begins to develop. This integration of self- and object representations constitutes the ego. The better such integration is carried out, the stronger the ego and the more differentiated it will be from the id.

The superego develops in a similar manner. However, rather than integrating self- and other representations, the superego integrates idealized and sadistic/persecutory representations of parental figures. The more complete and coherent this integration, the less harsh and unrealistic the superego will be.

The id consists, at this point, simply of that which has not been integrated. It is composed of all-good and all-bad self- and object representations that the ego has failed to integrate. This unintegrated id material is unavailable to consciousness. Failure to integrate is a result of relational experiences that make such integration seem dangerous. For example, a child with a mother who viciously punishes any hint of anger will try to avoid such feelings in relation to her and will not integrate them into his or her representation of her. A child whose mother is unpredictable has no basis for integration. Such an individual is prone to what Kernberg has termed splitting: rapid and profound mood changes that do not affect one another. The person may at one time show rage and hatred and at another show idealization and love toward one and the same person without one emotion affecting the emergence of the other and without any awareness of the contradictory nature of these alternating mood states. These irruptions of id processes into consciousness are characteristic of borderline personality disorder. If development proceeds positively, however, splitting seldom occurs. Representations of self and other do get integrated and become more available to awareness. Some representations, however, seem dangerous even in their integrated state. These partially integrated object representations are repressed and come to reside in the id, just as classical psychoanalysis has described. Oedipal issues—combinations of good (sexual) and bad (aggressive) object relations that are deemed dangerous—fall into this category. When all goes well, the id contains repressed object representations in dynamically unconscious form. In Kernberg's conception, repression is a developmentally advanced, late-arriving defense mechanism that is relatively adaptive. In the classical view, repression is primitive. In Kernberg's view, relatively integrated object representations are repressed. In the classical view, primitive wishes and their derivatives are repressed.

## Self Psychology

The final psychoanalytic model of the unconscious comes from self psychology. This model has been most explicitly fleshed out by Stolorow and Atwood (Atwood and Stolorow 1984; Stolorow and Atwood 1989; Stolorow et al. 1987, 1992), who have termed their understanding the *intersubjective model*. The two most recent and complete formulations of this model are those of Stolorow and Atwood (1989) and of Stolorow et al. (1992). Our explication is drawn largely from these two sources.

A basic premise of self psychology is that all psychological phenomena develop within what is termed an *intersubjective matrix*. That means that a person requires an interacting other in order to make meaning out of life, and that such meaning develops in the subjective experience of the interaction between the person and the interacting other.

There are, in this model, three kinds of unconscious: prereflective, dynamic, and unvalidated. The prereflective unconscious is based on the person's developing understanding of the world; the dynamic and the unvalidated unconscious depend on the reaction of important others to the developing person's emotional expression.

The *prereflective unconscious* contains the socially obtained principles through which the person organizes his or her world. It constrains and shapes the understanding and interpretations the person has and makes about his or her surround. If experiences cannot be assimilated into these structures, they are either distorted (so as to make them fit) or ignored (so that they will not have to fit). Since information is usually open to interpretation, all experiences are profoundly shaped by the prereflective unconscious. The name *prereflective* signifies the fact that this division of the mind contains unexamined assumptions or axioms concerning how the world operates. The existence of this type of functioning means that all of our experiences and perceptions are subjectively shaded and influenced by our prevailing biases.[1] Defensive styles

---

[1] This notion served as the starting point for a series of perception experiments—termed the "new look"—that flourished in the 1950s (Dixon 1971, 1981; Erdelyi 1974) and is now making a comeback (Bornstein and Pittman 1992).

can be seen as prereflective in that they structure the person's interpretation of experience.[2]

No conflict or pathology is inherent in the prereflective unconscious. Everyone must organize his or her experience according to some logic. People must give meaning to their experiences. Such meaning develops through interactions with the interpersonal environment. The prereflective unconscious does influence what can become conflictual, however, in that what a person finds safe or dangerous and even what she or he notices at all is constrained by its structure. It therefore constitutes the most basic unconscious division and underlies the other two types of unconscious described below.

The infant's developing consciousness is articulated through the validating responsiveness of the interpersonal environment, within the constraints of the prereflective unconscious—that is, a person's conscious experiential field expands to the degree that expression receives an affirmative response from important others in the environment. The more attuned the parental figure to the infant's expressions, the more those expressions are affirmed and the more the infant's range of conscious experience and mastery expand. The most critical experiences are those laden with affect, because they are the ones most open to interpretation and reflection. This conclusion is supported by Stern's (1985) work on affective attunement between mothers and their infants.

If the developing child's affective experiences are not validated or affirmed, the foundation is laid for evolution of the other two kinds of unconscious. When its affective expressions are ignored or rejected, the infant assumes that the parental figure is disapproving. This assumption generates a subjective feeling of danger and of conflict. The infant wishes to express and to integrate the affect but fears that doing so would jeopardize its tie with the parental figure. Because all of psychological organization and development depends on this tie, all of selfhood is thereby jeopard-

---

[2]In his classic book *Neurotic Styles*, Shapiro (1964) discussed some such defensive styles, although he termed them "neurotic."

ized. This is a traumatic experience for the developing child. Efforts at integration are therefore discontinued and the offending affect is walled off. Any feelings, memories, or other experiences that could potentially lead to the affect's expression suffer the same fate. By means of such repression, the dynamic unconscious is born and develops. Thus, the *dynamic unconscious* in this model consists of defensively walled-off affect states, as opposed to the drive derivatives of the classical model or the relationship configurations of object relations theory.

Finally, an infant need not have its affective expression ignored or rejected to be thwarted in its development. The environment may simply provide no opportunity for such expression. This occurs in situations of deprivation. The affective expression is not walled off; it simply never gets articulated in the first place. Such poorly developed affective expressions constitute the *unvalidated unconscious.*

Therapeutic technique is tailored to working with all three types of unconscious. The prereflective unconscious is the most important division since it underlies the others, and most analytic work is therefore directed toward illuminating it. The work involves bringing unquestioned assumptions into awareness so that the person can see how he or she structures the world and how this organization constrains his or her experiences.

The dynamic unconscious is treated by analyzing resistances. Resistance comes about because the person fears affective expression lest it result in destruction of interpersonal ties and, ultimately, in annihilation of the self. Articulation of experience is used to undo the deficits inherent in the unvalidated unconscious. Once such experiences are articulated, they will crystallize into a more organized structure.

Because all of psychological experience is said to take place within and be fostered by interpersonal interactions, the therapist–patient relationship assumes primary importance in self psychological approaches. Empathic understanding, seen as providing the validating responsiveness so needed by the patient, is the key technical variable. To be attuned to the patient is to help him or her. Interpretive activity is secondary.

The unconscious is also fuzzier in the self psychological model. What is conscious and what is unconscious shifts, depending on the intersubjective context. Such shifting between consciousness and unconsciousness is a product of the important other's responsiveness to and affirmation of different regions of the person's experiences. At first, the parental figure fills this role of important other. In therapy, it is the therapist. The relative constancy usually seen between what is conscious and what is unconscious is due to the self-fulfilling prophecy of the prereflective unconscious, the resistances of the dynamic unconscious, and the continued deprivation of the environment maintaining the unvalidated unconscious. To the extent that these factors shift, so does the boundary. Thus, unlike classical and object relations theory, self psychology specifies no clear difference between what is conscious and what is unconscious. Additionally, whereas in Stolorow's model the unconscious (like consciousness) is an intersubjective product, in the classical model it is intrapsychic.

## Comparing the Psychoanalytic Models

The models reviewed above differ enormously in their particulars. The classical model posits intrapsychic, relatively disembodied wishes and desires. Object relations theory sees wishes as connected to important others. Self psychology deals not with wishes but with interpersonal affect expression. The models also vary in their interpersonal emphases. The classical models barely acknowledge interpersonal issues, object relations theory views these issues as central, and self psychology construes them as all. The models likewise vary in terms of the qualitative differences between unconscious and conscious functioning. The topographical model posits the strongest distinction: the two are absolutely different. The structural model and object relations theory suggest that differences vary depending on organization. Self psychology sees virtually no differences between conscious and unconscious processing, only an ever-shifting boundary. In line with these qualitative differences, the topographical model posits very poor organization of unconscious processes. The structural and object relational models assert varying levels of organization. Self psychology postulates three organizational units ranging from very poorly organized (unvalidated) to very tightly organized (prereflective). Therapeutic goals and techniques according to the different models also vary, from bringing material into consciousness (topographical), to increasing organization through interpretation (structural and object relational), and finally to offering empathic understanding so as to foster development (self psychology).

So is there no point in discussing "the" psychoanalytic unconscious? Are the differences so great as to make this an impossible enterprise? The differences are great, it is true, but there are similarities as well. And these similarities serve to differentiate all of these psychoanalytic models from other conceptions of human functioning. First, unconscious processes are held to be central, nay primary, in all psychoanalytic conceptions. Next, these processes are affectively charged, and much of behavior is unconsciously motivated. Thus, *the psychoanalytic unconscious is centrally affective and motivational.* This means that it is largely irrational and that most of the origins of our behavior are unknown to us. Further, early experiences are critical to unconscious functioning. We become emotionally ill because of problems with unconscious functioning experienced at early, critical periods in our lives. Finally, although to varying degrees, depending on the model, empathic understanding and interpretation are the techniques that can help people overcome their unconsciously motivated problems (Josephs 1995).

## Cognitive Conceptions of the Unconscious

Early cognitive theorists (e.g., Neisser 1967) hypothesized that information was processed serially in stages. It soon became apparent, however, that such a hypothesis could not account for human information processing. Neuronal activity was simply too slow to allow for effective serial processing. Cognitivists now see the mind as composed of many relatively independent and specialized systems operating in parallel—that is, many things are going on at once. This concept has been termed *parallel distributed processing* (J. L. McClelland et al. 1986; Rumelhart et al. 1986). The mind is now seen as a hierarchy of parallel processors, each more or less independent of the others.

The information processed by the mind is transformed and then stored in associative networks. It is retrieved through activation of the appropriate associative network. The elements of some networks are very closely linked (i.e., the associations are extremely strong) such that activating any part of the network results in retrieval of all of its elements. Thus, the network functions as a unit. Such networks are termed *schemas.*

There are many types of schemas, categorized according to the type of information they contain and are applied to. Schemas powerfully influence the processing of new information by providing an organizing framework for such processing. To make experience intelligible, information is fit into existing schematic structures. Schemas are therefore strongly assimilative, in the Piagetian (Flavell 1963) sense. This means that the meaning of an experience can sometimes be distorted to fit schematic expectations.

Modern cognitive conceptions of unconscious processing derive from the notion of parallel processing. Because many things are going on in the mind simultaneously, they cannot all be conscious—that is, we cannot be aware of all of our parallel processing. In fact, most of it takes place outside of awareness. Such activity is most often referred to as implicit (cf. Reber 1992). Implicit processes constitute the cognitive unconscious. Some, like language acquisition (Chomsky 1957) and decision-making heuristics (Kahneman et al. 1982), are innate; others are developed through experience (Hasher and Zacks 1984). Cognitive psychologists have studied implicit memory (Schachter 1987), implicit perception (Kihlstrom 1990), implicit learning (Lewicki 1986; Reber 1992), and implicit knowledge (Nisbett and Wilson 1977). There have even been accounts of implicit motivation (D. C. McClelland et al. 1988; Weinberger and McClelland 1990).

Reviewers combing through these literatures have come to vastly different conclusions regarding the nature of unconscious processes. Greenwald (1992), in a featured *American Psychologist* paper, asserted that unconscious processes were simple and unsophisticated. He argued that such processes bear no resemblance whatsoever to psychoanalytic conceptions of unconscious processes. Kihlstrom (1990) also concluded that psychoanalytic conceptions were inaccurate. Yet Erdelyi (1985) has argued that psychoanalytic conceptions could be derived from cognitive conceptions. His book represents a brilliant translation of psychoanalysis into cognitive language. It thus appears that the cognitive literature is ambiguous and open to interpretation with regard to the nature of unconscious processes.

Few unified cognitive theories of the mind have been expounded; most of the work in this area is specialized and carried out in isolation (Reber 1992). Additionally, the work tends to focus on relatively simple, affectively neutral phenomena (Kihlstrom 1990; Weinberger, in press). A few exceptions exist (e.g., Cloitre, Chapter 3 in this volume), but they certainly do not constitute a central aspect of cognitive research. Extension of cognitive theories to clinical events or to psychoanalytic conceptions is therefore at a very preliminary stage. Much remains to be done (see Cloitre, Chapter 3 in this volume for serious efforts in this direction). We next review two cognitive models of the mind that we believe may be relevant to clinically meaningful unconscious processes: Baars' (1988a) "global workspace" theory and neodissociation theory (Hilgard 1986; Kihlstrom 1990, 1992).

## Global Workspace Theory

Global workspace theory (Baars 1988a) begins with the currently accepted cognitive notion of parallel distributed processing. The problem Baars attempts to address is how these specialized and often independent systems communicate with one another, for this they must do if experience and behavior are to demonstrate continuity and coherence. Baars posits what he terms a "central information exchange" as the medium for this communication. Many processors have access to this central exchange system, and it has outputs to virtually all of them. Once a mental system gains access to the central information exchange, the results of its processing become available to all of the other systems in the mind. This central information exchange is what we experience as consciousness. Thus, in one stroke, Baars has hypothesized a medium through which parallel distributed processes communicate and has explained the function of consciousness.

Baars sees the mind and its myriad of processors as akin to a group of specialized experts working independently on a problem. The only way they can let their colleagues know about the fruits of their labors is to publish them. Unlike the rest of us, however, they have but one outlet, the central information exchange (i.e., consciousness). Baars refers to this characterization as the "publicity metaphor" because consciousness makes results public to all members of the system.

In order for the messages to make sense, only one can be published at a time. This restriction accounts for the serial nature of consciousness. It also suggests the possibility of competition, as different outputs strive to attain consciousness. Baars has posited two means by which one output gains access to consciousness over others. The first has to do with strength of activation. The more strongly a system is activated, the more likely it is to be admitted into consciousness. We are more likely to notice a loud sound than soft whispering, all other things being equal.

All other things are not always equal, however, which brings us to the second factor controlling access to consciousness. Baars refers to this aspect as "context." In colloquial terms, context refers to the currently dominant state of mind. It is both the overarching umbrella under which processing takes place and the predominant goal of that processing. Context can be a mood. We are more likely to notice and to recall positive events when we are in a positive mood. Conversely, we are more likely to notice and to recall negative events when we are melancholy. Alternatively, context can be a major life goal such as becoming a lawyer. Would-be lawyers are more likely to become conscious of events relevant to their career choice than of other events. This is so even when they are not actively thinking about being lawyers. Would-be novelists would be more sensitive to characters around them, and so on. In such cases, a whisper may more easily achieve consciousness than a loud bang, if the right person is whispering.

If his hypotheses bear out, Baars' model would be a major advance in the history of the study of the mind. Baars is not particularly interested in clinical phenomena, however, although he believes that the model can account for such phenomena (Baars 1988b). Contexts are typically unconscious, even though they strongly influence what becomes conscious. Our patients would be better understood if we knew the contexts under which they are operating. Baars has suggested projective tests (e.g., sentence completion) as a way of reaching these unconscious contexts. He posits that repression involves one set of goals winning out over another in the competition for consciousness. The defeated goals are then dissociated but still contribute to context. It is not clear exactly how such choices are made or how defeated goals contribute to context in Baars' model. It might require someone with more of a clinical interest than Baars to make these connections. At present, global workspace theory can provide only tantalizing hints about clinical phenomena.

## Neodissociation Theory

Neodissociation theory has clearer links to clinical phenomena than does global workspace theory. In fact, it has a pedigree just as long and distinguished as that of psychoanalysis. Neodissociation theory can be traced back to Janet (Ellenberger 1970; Hilgard 1973), a contemporary of Freud. Here we briefly review Janet's views (see Weinberger, in preparation, for a more complete explication) and then discuss Hilgard's (1986, 1992) extension of this theory.

According to Janet, the mind is composed of a myriad of complex, goal-oriented activities, each possessed of a rudimentary consciousness. Janet termed these elements of the mind *automatisms* (Kihlstrom 1984). Under optimal circumstances, all automatisms are integrated by consciousness. Sometimes, however, due to inadequate resources and/or traumatic stress, integration fails to take place. When this occurs, the relevant automatisms are split off or dissociated from consciousness; however, they continue to function outside of awareness and voluntary control—in Janet's terminology, they are "subconscious." Hypnosis is an artificial means of causing and mending such dissociations. Dissociation is inherently pathological in Janet's system. It is the therapist's task to restore health by helping the person integrate (i.e., bring into consciousness) the dissociated automatisms.

Janet's views, although influential for a time, rapidly lost their popularity as Freud's views became known. By the mid-1960s, references to dissociation had all but disappeared from the literature (Hilgard 1973). Two related factors combined to bring Janet's views back into the mainstream. The first of these was Hilgard's neodissociation theory (Hilgard 1986, 1992); the second was the cognitive notion of parallel distributed processing.

Hilgard's (1986) model took as its point of departure the observation that apparently planned and effortful behavior often proceeds outside of awareness. Such behavior is seen as dissociated from consciousness. To account for these phenomena, Hilgard posited a hierarchy of systems in the mind topped by a central regulatory mechanism. This central regulator represents consciousness. The hierarchy is flexible and shifts often. It is up to the central regulatory mechanism to monitor and control the actions of the subsystems in this hierarchy—that is, the central regulatory mechanism has executive and monitoring functions. Thus, the function of consciousness is to control and monitor the subsystems of the mind. Each subsystem also has its own executive and monitoring functions. The subsystems thus have a rudimentary kind of consciousness.

The central system and its subsystems are not always in communication. Hilgard discovered this circumstance by way of the phenomenon of the "hidden observer." It turns out that hypnotized subjects told not to feel, or see, or whatever, nonetheless continue to monitor their subjective experiences. Thus, a hypnotized subject told to plunge his hand into cold water without feeling it will do so with no outward sign of discomfort. However, if the subject is asked to rate his pain, he will be able to do so with little difficulty. The monitoring function thus remains intact. What has happened, says Hilgard, is that the links to the executive function of the central regulatory mechanism (i.e., phenomenal consciousness) have been temporarily derailed. The hypnotist has taken over the executive function. The person's subsystems still operate, however, and can report to the hypnotist, much as they ordinarily report to consciousness. Such dissociations are ubiquitous in normal life, as evidenced by people doing two things at once, only one of which they are aware, or doing something with no awareness whatsoever. Hilgard differs from Janet, who saw dissociation as abnormal, in this regard (cf. Fromm 1992).

Hilgard developed his model before the advent of the notion of parallel distributed processing. It fits in beautifully with that model of the mind, however, and so was quite prescient (cf. Kihlstrom 1992). The subsystems can be equated with the parallel processors. This correspondence has added to the popularity of Hilgard's model and to its extension by thinkers such as Kihlstrom (1992). Kihlstrom has expanded the scope of neodissociation theory to account for much of cognitive behavior. For example, he has suggested that some subsystems, such as language skills and feature detectors, are never linked to the central regulatory mechanism. Links between systems are sometimes severed—for example, when a skill is so well learned that it becomes automatic (Hasher and Zacks 1984). Reading represents such a skill. On occasion, stimulation is so weak that the conscious system is never affected, although various subsystems are; this is what occurs when subliminal events (implicit perception) affect behavior (Bornstein and Pittman 1992). Neurological damage can physically sever the links between systems. Thus, persons with anterograde amnesia often show evidence of implicit memory when asked to complete a word fragment (Schachter 1987). Individuals with prosopagnosia (inability to recognize faces) nonetheless exhibit differential responsiveness to old and new faces (De Haan et al. 1987). Kihlstrom (1990) and Reber (1992) have summarized these phenomena.

All of the phenomena described above can be seen as dissociated, and all are unconscious to some degree. Kihlstrom (1987) discussed these phenomena in terms of their level of consciousness, thereby lending more specificity to the model. He described three types of unconscious or dissociated experiences:

1. The first is *truly unconscious;* it can never be directly known introspectively but only inferred. The clearest example of such an experience is innate procedural knowledge (e.g., the phonological and linguistic principles through which we decode speech). Learned procedural knowledge can be made conscious only with great effort and often at the cost of efficiency (e.g., musicianship). (Although it seems to us that such routinized activity is not strictly unconscious in the sense of not being open to introspection, we will follow Kihlstrom's convention and categorize it as he does.)
2. The second level of consciousness, termed *preconscious,* involves declarative knowledge that has not been activated strongly enough to achieve phenomenal awareness. Such mental contents are latent, requiring only the attainment of a certain threshold to be conscious. Procedural knowledge can interact with such latent declarative knowledge to produce preconscious structures. This is what happens in subliminal perception, for example. The subliminal stimulation is processed even though it is not strong enough to reach phenomenal awareness.
3. Finally, Kihlstrom discusses a *subconscious* level of awareness (after Janet's use of the term) in which the stimulation is above threshold but the person is still not aware of it. Examples of this level of awareness are hypnotic states and clinical dissociative phenomena. Such subconscious phenomena represent a major puzzle for cognitive conceptions of the mind. They imply that high levels of activation are not sufficient to produce conscious awareness. Kihlstrom (1990, 1992) solves this problem by hypothesizing that awareness requires a connection to a representation of the self. Thus, *unconscious processes can be described as those not linked to the self-system or self-schema.* Some experiences (e.g., subliminal stimuli) are too weak to make contact with the self-system. Others are preempted (e.g., through hyp-

nosis) or are actively prevented from reaching the system (e.g., traumatic memories). And still others simply cannot reach the system because of the way we are wired up. If the self-schema is identified with the executive and monitoring functions described by Hilgard, we have a working model of consciousness and unconsciousness. Experiences that do not make contact with this superordinate (self or executive) system are unconscious; those that do are conscious.

Different types of phenomena are variably likely to connect to self-representations: procedural knowledge (the truly unconscious) virtually never connects; preconscious experiences connect only if they are activated strongly enough; and subconscious experiences require special procedures.

Neodissociation theory has several clinical applications. Obsessive-compulsive behavior can be conceptualized as a manifestation of weak central executive control in combination with an intact central monitor. Thus, the patient is fully aware and critical of the pathological nature of his or her thoughts and/or behavior but is unable to stop them (Hilgard 1992). A sociopathic person may have intact executive functioning but inadequate critical (monitoring) faculties. Conflict of any sort may be conceptualized as an imbalance between executive and monitoring functions. Negative hallucinations and amnesia can be understood as a dissociation between subsystems and the executive self-system. The flashbacks of posttraumatic stress disorder may be a product of memories dissociated from the self-system (Kihlstrom 1992). Implicit memories may also account for the apparently inexplicable fears and vague forebodings of abuse victims (Cloitre, Chapter 3 in this volume). And finally, dissociative identity disorder may result from the development of two or more executive self-systems linked to the same subordinate subsystems (Kihlstrom 1992). But although neodissociation theory can account for many clinical observations, it is notably silent as to what to do about them. Presumably, the dissociations must be mended, possibly through connection with the self-system; however, we have read of no clinical techniques for doing so. Although it is possible to speculate on what treatment would look like in this model, few clinical or research data are available as yet.[3]

## Comparing the Psychoanalytic and the Cognitive Conceptions

There are some similarities between cognitive and psychoanalytic views of unconscious processing. Both see unconscious processing as important and as constituting a significant portion of mental functioning. Both see some qualitative differences between conscious and unconscious processing. Both see unconscious processing as more primitive and less malleable than conscious processing.

There are also some very profound differences between the two. Most importantly, their databases and central constructs are radically different. Psychoanalytic views on unconscious processing (like all of psychoanalytic theory) were built upon and, to a large degree, continue to be based on extensive clinical observations. The psychoanalytic research base is notoriously poor. The research programs of Shevrin and colleagues (e.g., Shevrin et al. 1992) and of Silverman (e.g., Silverman 1976; Silverman and Weinberger 1985) provide the exceptions that prove the rule. Cognitive conceptions tend to be rigorously empirical; much of the work is laboratory based. But it rarely examines clinically meaningful phenomena.

The complementary nature of the strengths and weaknesses of psychoanalysis and cognitive science might suggest that the two would be perfect marriage partners. Each could provide what the other lacks, and the resulting union could explain much of human mental (and specifically unconscious) functioning. Horowitz (1988b) has embarked upon a program to do just that. He has made use of schema theory to elucidate self- and object representations while retaining the biological drives of classical theory.

---

[3]Of course, there is the immense literature on cognitive therapy (see Hollon and Beck 1994 for a comprehensive review). Surprisingly, however, it has little to say about unconscious processes.

Stein (1992, Chapter 6 in this volume) has offered similar notions. Erdelyi (1985) has shown that experimental cognitive findings can fit with psychoanalytic observations. Cloitre (Chapter 3 in this volume) has applied experimental cognitive findings on unconscious processes to the study of specific clinical populations. A recent workshop held by the National Institute of Mental Health (Kurtzman, in press) was devoted to integrating cognitive science and psychoanalysis.

So is this the solution? Can the psychoanalytic unconscious be understood by means of cognitive conceptions? Greenwald (1992) and Kihlstrom (1990) say no; Erdelyi (1985), Horowitz (1988b), and Stein (1992, Chapter 6 in this volume) say yes. So it is our guess that the answer is maybe. But we wish to sound a caution. Even if it were theoretically possible to understand psychoanalysis in cognitive terms, such efforts may be premature. Cognitive science is built upon a nonaffective model of the mind. Its very name, "cognitive science," is indicative of its lack of focus on affect. Whereas the terms *affect, emotion,* and *motivation* are almost entirely absent from the cognitive science literature (Weinberger, in press; Weinberger and McClelland 1990), these terms are absolutely central to psychoanalytic conceptions. We cannot assume that a science almost exclusively devoted to emotionless functioning can be employed to shed light on passion and psychopathology.

An analogy to the study of memory may make our position clearer. Ebbinghaus (1885/1964) began his experimental study of memory by memorizing lists of nonsense syllables. He did this because he wished to isolate the laws of memory from what he saw as the confounding variables of meaning and emotional involvement. His work generated replicable and valid laws. But as Bartlett (1932) pointed out, meaning is a critical aspect of memory. We cannot understand memory without it. Once meaningful memory began to be studied, a whole new set of laws appeared (Solso 1988). In many cases, these laws were qualitatively different from those of Ebbinghaus.

The unconscious events we see in our patients are often imbued with affect and importance. For the most part, cognitive researchers have chosen not to examine such variables (cf. Kihlstrom 1990; Shevrin et al. 1992; Weinberger, in press; Weinberger and McClelland 1990). It may be that information processing of emotionally meaningful and important stimuli is qualitatively different from that of affectively neutral stimuli. There are already hints that this is so. Reiman et al. (1989) have shown that the neural systems underlying affect and cognition are quite different. Posner and Rothbart (1989) have argued that affective systems have their own neural bases and operating rules. Shevrin and colleagues (e.g., 1992) demonstrated that subliminal stimuli evocative of unconscious conflict showed a different pattern of evoked potential in the brain than either supraliminal stimulation or subliminal presentation of ordinary unpleasant words or even of words consciously related to the conflict. And finally, subliminal psychodynamic activation, developed by Silverman and others (Hardaway 1990; Silverman 1976; Silverman and Weinberger 1985; Weinberger and Hardaway 1990), shows that subliminal stimulation of psychoanalytically derived, emotionally laden messages affects subsequent behavior in a way that stimulation of neutral messages does not.

Until we systematically compare affectively meaningful with affectively neutral stimuli, we should not uncritically accept cognitive notions of the unconscious. By the same token, until we empirically examine psychoanalytic propositions in a systematic and rigorous fashion, we should not uncritically accept psychoanalytic notions of the unconscious.

We propose a different marriage than that suggested by psychoanalytically sympathetic cognitivists. We do not think that cognitive explanations should be uncritically applied to psychoanalytic ideas. Such a strategy carries the danger, detailed above, of improper generalization. We suggest, instead, that cognitive science incorporate the type of affect-laden stimuli stressed by psychoanalysis (e.g., love, sexuality, aggression, guilt, passion, competition). Thus, we recommend the use of cognitive science *methods* to test psychoanalytic ideas. Such an approach would provide both the rigor so lacking in psychoanalysis and the affective focus so missing in cognitive science. And then, let the chips fall where they may.

# References

Arlow JA, Brenner C: Psychoanalytic Concepts and the Structural Theory. New York, International Universities Press, 1964

Atwood G, Stolorow R: Structures of Subjectivity: Explorations in Psychoanalytic Phenomenology. Hillsdale, NJ, Analytic Press, 1984

Baars BJ: A Cognitive Theory of Consciousness. New York, Cambridge University Press, 1988a

Baars BJ: Momentary forgetting as a "resetting" of a conscious global workspace due to competition between incompatible contexts, in Psychodynamics and Cognition. Edited by Horowitz MJ. Chicago, IL, University of Chicago Press, 1988b, pp 269–293

Bartlett FC: Remembering: A Study in Experimental and Social Psychology. Cambridge, UK, Cambridge University Press, 1932

Bornstein RF, Pittman TS (eds): Perception Without Awareness. New York, Guilford, 1992

Brenner C: The Mind in Conflict. New York, International Universities Press, 1982

Chomsky N: Syntactic Structures. The Hague, Netherlands, Mouton, 1957

De Haan EHF, Young AW, Newcombe F: Face recognition without awareness. Cognitive Neuropsychology 4:385–415, 1987

Dixon NF: Subliminal Perception: The Nature of a Controversy. New York, McGraw-Hill, 1971

Dixon NF: Preconscious Processing. New York, Wiley, 1981

Ebbinghaus H: Memory. Translated by Ruger HA, Bussenius CE. New York, Dover, 1964 (original work published in 1885)

Ellenberger HF: The Discovery of the Unconscious: The History and Evolution of Dynamic Psychiatry. New York, Basic Books, 1970

Erdelyi MH: A new look at the New Look: perceptual defense and vigilance. Psychol Rev 81:1–25, 1974

Erdelyi MH: Psychoanalysis: Freud's Cognitive Psychology. New York, WH Freeman, 1985

Fairbairn WD: Theoretical and experimental aspects of psycho-analysis. Br J Med Psychol 25:122–127, 1952

Flavell JH: The Developmental Psychology of Jean Piaget. New York, Van Nostrand, 1963

Freud S: The interpretation of dreams (1900), in The Standard Edition of the Complete Psychological Works of Sigmund Freud, Vols 4 and 5. Translated and edited by Strachey J. London, Hogarth Press, 1953

Freud S: The unconscious (1915), in The Standard Edition of the Complete Psychological Works of Sigmund Freud, Vol 14. Translated and edited by Strachey J. London, Hogarth Press, 1957, pp 159–215

Freud S: The ego and the id (1923), in The Standard Edition of the Complete Psychological Works of Sigmund Freud, Vol 19. Translated and edited by Strachey J. London, Hogarth Press, 1961, pp 3–68

Freud S: The loss of reality in neurosis and psychosis (1924), in The Standard Edition of the Complete Psychological Works of Sigmund Freud, Vol 19. Translated and edited by Strachey J. London, Hogarth Press, 1961, pp 181–187

Freud S: Beyond the pleasure principle (1920), in The Standard Edition of the Complete Psychological Works of Sigmund Freud, Vol 18. Translated and edited by Strachey J. London, Hogarth Press, 1955, pp 1–64

Freud S: Inhibitions, symptoms and anxiety (1926), in The Standard Edition of the Complete Psychological Works of Sigmund Freud, Vol 20. Translated and edited by Strachey J. London, Hogarth Press, 1959, pp 75–175

Freud S: Splitting of the ego in the process of defence (1940 [1938]), in The Standard Edition of the Complete Psychological Works of Sigmund Freud, Vol 23. Translated and edited by Strachey J. London, Hogarth Press, 1964, pp 271–278

Fromm E: Dissociation, repression, cognition, and voluntarism. Consciousness and Cognition 1:40–46, 1992

Greenberg JR, Mitchell SA: Object Relations in Psychoanalytic Theory. Cambridge, MA, Harvard University Press, 1983

Greenwald AG: New look 3: unconscious cognition reclaimed. Am Psychol 47:766–779, 1992

Hardaway R: Subliminally activated symbiotic fantasies: facts and artifacts. Psychol Bull 107:177–195, 1990

Hasher L, Zacks RT: Automatic processing of fundamental information. Am Psychol 39:1372–1388, 1984

Hilgard ER: Dissociation revisited, in Historical Conceptions of Psychology. Edited by Henle M, Jaynes J, Sullivan J. New York, Springer, 1973, pp 205–219

Hilgard ER: Divided Consciousness: Multiple Controls in Human Thought and Action, Revised Edition. New York, Wiley, 1986

Hilgard ER: Divided consciousness and dissociation. Consciousness and Cognition 1:16–31, 1992

Hollon SD, Beck AT: Cognitive and cognitive-behavioral therapies, in Handbook of Psychotherapy and Behavior Change, 4th Edition. Edited by Bergin AE, Garfield SL. New York, Wiley, 1994, pp 467–508

Horowitz MJ: Introduction to Psychodynamics: A New Synthesis. New York, Basic Books, 1988a

Horowitz MJ: Psychodynamic phenomena and their explanation, in Psychodynamics and Cognition. Edited by Horowitz MJ. Chicago, IL, University of Chicago Press, 1988b, pp 3–20

Josephs L: Balancing Empathy and Interpretation. Northvale, NJ, Jason Aronson, 1995

Kahneman D, Slovic P, Tversky A (eds): Judgment Under Uncertainty: Heuristics and Biases. New York, Cambridge University Press, 1982

Kernberg O: Borderline Conditions and Pathological Narcissism. New York, Jason Aronson, 1975

Kernberg O: Object Relations Theory and Clinical Psychoanalysis. New York, Jason Aronson, 1976

Kernberg O: Self, ego, effects and drives. J Am Psychoanal Assoc 30:893–915, 1981

Kernberg O: The dynamic unconscious and the self, in Theories of the Unconscious and Theories of the Self. Edited by Stern R. Hillsdale, NJ, Analytic Press, 1987, pp 3–25

Kihlstrom JF: Conscious, subconscious, unconscious: a cognitive perspective, in The Unconscious Reconsidered. Edited by Bowers KS, Meichenbaum D. New York, Wiley, 1984, pp 149–211

Kihlstrom JF: The cognitive unconscious. Science 237:1445–1452, 1987

Kihlstrom JF: The psychological unconscious, in The Handbook of Personality. Edited by Pervin H. New York, Guilford, 1990, pp 445–464

Kihlstrom JF: Dissociation and dissociations: a comment on consciousness and cognition. Consciousness and Cognition 1:47–53, 1992

Kurtzman H (ed): Integrating Cognitive Science and Psychoanalysis. London, Oxford University Press (in press)

Lewicki P: Processing information about covariations that cannot be articulated. J Exp Psychol Learn Mem Cogn 12:135–146, 1986

McClelland DC, Koestner RF, Weinberger J: How do self-attributed and implicit motives differ? Psychol Rev 96:690–702, 1988

McClelland JL, Rumelhart DE, PDP Research Group (eds): Parallel Distributed Processing: Explorations in the Microstructure of Cognition, Vol 2: Psychological and Biological Models. Cambridge, MA, MIT Press, 1986

Neisser U: Cognitive Psychology. New York, Appleton-Century-Crofts, 1967

Nisbett RE, Wilson TD: Telling more than we can know: verbal reports on mental processes. Psychol Rev 84:231–259, 1977

Posner MI, Rothbart MK: Intentional chapters on unintended thoughts, in Unintended Thought. Edited by Uleman JS, Bargh JA. New York, Guilford, 1989, pp 450–469

Rapaport D: The structure of psychoanalytic theory (Psychological Issues 2, monograph 6). New York, International Universities Press, 1960

Reber AS: The cognitive unconscious: an evolutionary perspective. Consciousness and Cognition 1:93–133, 1992

Reich W: Character Analysis (1933). New York, Pocket Books, 1976

Reiman EM, Fusselman MJ, Fox PT, et al: Activation of temporopolar cortex in the production of anticipatory anxiety. Science 243:1071–1074, 1989

Rumelhart DE, McClelland JL, PDP Research Group (eds): Parallel Distributed Processing: Explorations in the Microstructure of Cognition, Vol 1: Foundations. Cambridge, MA, MIT Press, 1986

Schachter DL: Implicit memory: history and current status. J Exp Psychol Learn Mem Cogn 13:501–518, 1987

Shapiro D: Neurotic Styles. New York, Basic Books, 1964

Shevrin H, Williams WJ, Marshall RE, et al: Event-related potential indicators of the dynamic unconscious. Consciousness and Cognition 1:340–366, 1992

Silverman LH: Psychoanalytic theory: the reports of my death are greatly exaggerated. Am Psychol 31:621–637, 1976

Silverman LH, Weinberger J: Mommy and I are one: implications for psychotherapy. Am Psychol 40:1296–1308, 1985

Solso RL: Cognitive Psychology, 2nd Edition. Newton, MA, Allyn & Bacon, 1988

Stein DJ: Psychoanalysis and cognitive science: contrasting models of the mind. J Am Acad Psychoanal 20:543–555, 1992

Stern DN: The Interpersonal World of the Infant. New York, Basic Books, 1985

Stolorow RD, Atwood GE: The unconscious and unconscious fantasy: an intersubjective-developmental perspective. Psychoanalytic Inquiry 9:364–374, 1989

Stolorow RD, Brandschaft B, Atwood G: Psychoanalytic Treatment: An Intersubjective Approach. Hillsdale, NJ, Analytic Press, 1987

Stolorow RD, Atwood GE, Brandschaft B: Three realms of the unconscious and their therapeutic transformation. Psychoanalytic Rev 79:25–30, 1992

Weinberger J: Unconscious Processes. New York, Guilford (in preparation)

Weinberger J, Hardaway R: Separating science from myth in subliminal psychodynamic activation. Clinical Psychology Review 10:727–756, 1990

Weinberger J, McClelland DC: Cognitive versus traditional motivational models: irreconcilable or complementary? in Handbook of Motivation and Cognition, Vol 2. Edited by Higgins ET, Sorrentino RM. New York, Guilford, 1990, pp 562–597

Weinberger J, Siegel P, De Camello A: What kind of integration do we want? in Integrating Cognitive Science and Psychoanalysis. Edited by Kurtzman H. London, Oxford University Press (in press)

Chapter 3

# Conscious and Unconscious Memory: A Model of Functional Amnesia

Marylene Cloitre, Ph.D.

## Introduction and Historical Overview

An often-cited example (Cloitre 1992; Ellenberger 1970; Schachter 1987; Tobias et al. 1992) of knowledge without awareness is a case reported by Pierre Janet (1893) concerning a woman with functional amnesia for a traumatic event in which she was mistakenly informed by a messenger at her door that her husband had died. Although the woman had no conscious recollection of the event, she nonetheless "froze with terror" whenever she passed the door the man had entered. This example is one of many reported cases in which an individual demonstrates affective, motor-sensory, or behavioral knowledge of a traumatic event of which he or she has no conscious recollection (Ellenberger 1970; Freud 1894/1962; Terr 1994). The phenomenon that an individual can be in a state of "knowing and not knowing" (Erdelyi 1985), apparently so familiar to clinicians, had posed a vexing if not impossible paradox to philosophers and psychologists in the first half of the 20th century. The paradox appeared so unwieldy that scientists often either rejected these observations as theoretically impossible and as misconstruals of some other phenomenon or simply ignored the reports altogether.

This paradox became conceptually tenable in the early 1960s with the advent of computer technology. Computers provided the blueprint for a new conceptualization of mental functioning. In computer systems, information could be stored in independent but interacting modules, each of which might have partial or no knowledge of the contents of the other modules; intermodule access to information could be governed by an executive system that oversaw the operations of the parts. If computers could do this, why not that presumably more complex processing system, the human mind? Abstract arguments about the logical impossibility of a state of "knowing and not knowing" dissolved in the face of a technical feat that realized exactly this paradox.

Since the mid-1980s, several studies of clinical and nonclinical populations have shown that knowledge without awareness is a relatively common phenomenon and that experiences not available to consciousness nevertheless influence perception, judgment, and action (Bowers 1984; Kihlstrom 1987; J. M. G. Williams et al. 1988). This variety of phenomena can be represented as part of the implicit/explicit memory distinction now so frequently studied among cognitive scientists. *Explicit memory* refers to conscious recollection of information to which a person is exposed, and *implicit memory* characterizes those situations in which information "encoded during a particular episode is subsequently expressed without conscious or deliberate recollection" (Schachter 1987, p. 501). Several studies have demonstrated that these two forms of memory are relatively dissociable or independent and that this dissociation seems linked to differences in the kinds of information carried by or expressed in these types of memory. Whereas explicit memory is formed by and relies on the meaningful elaboration of events and their relationship to other information in the memory network (i.e., is "conceptually driven"), implicit memory is most often expressed by behaviors that depend on exposure to and processing of sensory-perceptual or motor aspects of experience (i.e., is "data driven") (see Richardson-Klavehn and Bjork 1988; Roediger et al. 1989).

Perhaps the earliest known description of an implicit/explicit memory dissociation was reported by Claparède (1911/1951) in connection with a neurological case of amnesia (see Schachter 1987). Claparède (1911/1951) described an amnesic woman who hesitated to shake hands with him after he had pricked her with a pin during a handshake, although she had no recollection of him or the handshake. The memory dissociation is demonstrated by the fact that although the woman's behavior was influenced by the event, she had no conscious recollection of it.

From a behavioral perspective, hysterical, or functional, amnesia can be characterized as an instance of dissociation between explicit and implicit memory in which conscious, or explicit, memory for an event is not—or is only partially—available but implicit memory is intact. The behavior of the amnesic woman described by Janet shows many parallels to that of the woman in Claparède's case. The impairment of explicit memory is reflected by the fact that the woman had no conscious recollection of the upsetting episode by the doorway. Implicit memory is apparent from her emotion-laden behavior (fear and terror) when presented with a visual cue (the doorway) that represented one aspect of the initial experience. In both cases, an emotional response was elicited by the presence of a visual cue associated with the affectively laden memory, despite the absence of any conscious recollection of the event.

Of course, the source or mechanisms of the amnesia are clear for the neurological but not the functional case of amnesia. The patient with neurological amnesia has a lesion or some organic disorder that prevents him or her from having conscious recollection of most experiences. In contrast, no ready explanation exists for the dissociation between explicit and implicit memory observed in functional amnesia.

## Requirements for a Cognitive Model of Functional Amnesia

My goal in this chapter is to elucidate the characteristics of the implicit/explicit memory distinction and to assess the extent to which this framework provides a useful context in which to conceptualize and test the nature of functional amnesia. To provide a satisfactory description of functional amnesia, the implicit/explicit memory distinction must have at least three features. First, implicit and explicit memory must be shown to be dissociable in a way that is applicable to the experience of the neurologically intact individual with functional amnesia: it must allow for the absence of conscious awareness of an event and the simultaneous expression of knowledge of the event through some other behavior. Second, the knowledge the functionally amnesic person expresses concerning the "forgotten" event is often of a somatic or affective nature—thus, implicit memory must be shown to have motor or sensory-perceptual characteristics. Last and perhaps most important, some *psychological* mechanism must be specified in the model that can produce functional (i.e., nonorganic and reversible) amnesia for events within the domain of explicit memory but leave implicit memory unaffected.

The issue of the source and mechanisms of functional amnesia has, of course, a long history, dominated by Freud's notion of repression and Janet's notion of dissociation. Beyond the contentiousness of psychologists and philosophers concerning the paradox of "both knowing and not knowing," there was for them something repellent, displeasing, or simply unassimilable about the idea of repression (see Bjork 1989; Holmes 1974), and thus the notion of the unconscious was frequently rejected on the more concrete grounds that no acceptable mechanism for understanding this concept existed within the purview of cognitive science. Nevertheless, two bridges can be constructed between the specific observations of Freud and Janet—namely, purposeful or motivated forgetting and the assumptions of cognitive science.

## The Cognitive Science of Freud

Freud's initial characterization of functional amnesia was based on the reports of patients who could explicitly recall conscious efforts to "push away," "not think about," or in some way "suppress" an emotionally painful idea, memory, or experience (Freud 1894/ 1962). As noted by Erdelyi and Goldberg (1979), Freud related an exchange he had with one of his patients, Miss Lucy R., that provides evidence of this view. He asked her, "if you knew you loved your employee, why didn't you tell me?"; to which she responded, "I didn't know or rather I did not want to know. I wanted to drive it out of my head and not think of it again: and I believe lately I have succeeded" (Breuer and Freud 1893/1955, p. 117).

According to Freud, these intentional efforts of forgetting were the result not only of the patient's encounter with a painful idea but also of her evaluation that she lacked the power to resolve the dilemma by the "processes of thought" (Freud 1894/1962, p. 69). Thus, such "forgetting" appears to be essentially an effort to flee from psychic pain when other mental efforts are deemed unlikely to succeed in resolving the emotional disturbance. This type of response to the internal objects of the psychic world (ideas and/or emotions) can be viewed as parallel to the phenomenon observed in the external world—the fight-or-flight response in the face of an impending threat. If an individual feels that he or she is unable to successfully fight off an encroaching threat, the alternative survival response is to flee from the threat. Viewed in this way, functional amnesia is an adaptation to perceived dangers in the psychic world. It is also a parsimonious explanation of human motivation, as it suggests that the desire to avoid threat or pain cuts across both the cognitive and the behavioral domains of human experience.

The notion of functional amnesia as an adaptive strategy intended to ensure the functioning of the organism actually fits rather well with certain information-processing ideas of current cognitive science. One of the basic principles of the information-processing perspective is that humans select out and attend to only a subset of the rich and varied amount of information available in the environment. This selective process is considered to represent an adaptation to the discrepancy between the finite capacities humans have to process information and the nearly infinite amount of information available in the environment. It is believed that the basic purpose of the selection process is to organize information, make experience comprehensible, and thus facilitate goal-directed behavior.

Cognitive scientists have not typically considered the role of emotions in the operation of selective processing. However, it would not seem unreasonable that humans would enlist all resources at their disposal to aid them in selecting information that would maximize their functioning in the environment. Avoiding an emotionally troubling memory or any information in the environment associated with the memory could minimize psychic distress or maximize psychic well-being and thus contribute to successful goal-directed functioning. This view of amnesia fits well within a functional analysis of selective processing.

For the reasons articulated above, it is suggested that functional amnesia can be viewed as selective memory in the service of adaptation to the (internal and/or external) environment. Interestingly, some of Pierre Janet's ideas about consciousness, the subconscious, and environmental adaptation, at least as described by modern thinkers (Perry and Laurence 1984), are remarkably consistent with this suggestion.

## The Cognitive Science of Janet

Janet proposed that ideally, humans could be consciously aware of all experiences—from automatic responses to sensory percepts to the higher and more complex activities involved in the synthesis and organization of such percepts. According to Janet, the purpose of the organization and synthesis of percepts was to help the individual adapt to his or her environment and function in a healthful manner. Consciousness was viewed as a process of continual scanning across a field of sensations, perceptions, and memories. Janet suggested that when some type of psychic pain occurred in relation to a percept, the organism withdrew consciousness from this area of perceptual-synthetic activity in order to conserve energy. This restriction of consciousness can be viewed rather concretely as the narrowing of a spotlight over the activities and events of the internal world. The elements excluded from this purview are not synthesized into the mainstream of conscious experience but rather become dissociated or disaggregated from it, forming what Janet called the subconscious and Freud later called the unconscious. As a result of this disaggregation, an individual could develop and exhibit two alternating sets of memories. Janet believed that restoring equilibrium to the organism required bringing the disaggregated material into the focus of consciousness and integrating it with the mainstream flux of feelings, ideas, and sensations.

Janet's notions about the processes by which memories are lost to conscious awareness are consistent with current cognitive science notions of selective attention and memory. For example, the idea of a "restriction of consciousness" as an adaptive response to psychic pain is similar to current cognitive science notions of an attentional "spotlight" on the memory field and the more general theoretical assumption of the adaptive character of the human information-processing system. Interestingly, Janet viewed the formation of the subconscious as a pathological phenomenon that did not occur among healthy individuals. In this regard, current empirical literature does not support Janet. Rather, implicit memory, the cognitive science analogue of the subconscious, is a form of memory that is biologically given, occurs in the behaviors of all humans, and expresses both pathological and nonpathological phenomena.

## Summary

In this chapter, I present a selective review of the literature on the implicit/explicit memory distinction as it contributes to the development of a model of functional amnesia. Each section of the chapter describes studies that support one of the points needed to develop the model: 1) the dissociable nature of implicit and explicit memory, 2) the perceptual-sensory nature of implicit memory, 3) selective aspects of conscious memory, and 4) differential selectivity in explicit and implicit memory. This discussion is followed by application of the model to the assessment of memory functioning among persons who have experienced traumatic events—in particular, childhood abuse—and a broader discussion of the role of cognitive science in the study of traumatic memories of early-life abuse.

# The Dissociable Nature of Implicit and Explicit Memory

Several studies have shown that factors influencing explicit memory performance are quite different from those influencing implicit memory. The dissociation in performances on these two types of memory tasks has led to the suggestion that implicit and explicit memory are distinct and relatively independent memory systems or processes. The most typical dissociative phenomena observed are the ease with which, and the various means by which, explicit memory for an event becomes impaired, whereas under the same conditions implicit memory remains intact.

As previously mentioned, Claparède (1911/1951) provided one of the earliest descriptions of an implicit/explicit memory dissociation in his case report of a woman with neurologically induced amnesia. Systematic studies of neurologically impaired individuals conducted by Schachter and others (see Schachter 1987) have consistently found that amnesic individuals are seriously impaired on standard tests of explicit memory but perform at normal levels on a variety of implicit memory tasks.

Amnesic individuals demonstrate intact implicit memory for many tasks that depend on the motor-perceptual or sensory aspects of experience. Despite their inability to recall ever having performed certain tasks, persons with amnesia exhibit exposure-related performance facilitation in activities such as perceptual identification of briefly flashed or degraded words, reading of mirror-inverted script, serial pattern learning, and puzzle solving (see Schachter 1987). Another interesting characteristic of the dissociation observed in amnesic persons is that implicit—but not explicit—memory persists for the evaluative or affective aspects of experience. Johnson et al. (1985) found that when presented with photographs of men, individuals with amnesia produced positive or negative evaluations consistent with evaluatively loaded biographies recounted earlier about the men, although they did not recognize the men or have any conscious recollection of ever having seen the photographs before.

Experimental and pharmacological manipulations in non–neurologically impaired subjects have also produced dissociation of implicit and explicit memory. It has been consistently found that variations in the degree of elaborative or meaningful analysis of a target event have a significant effect on explicit memory tasks but do not influence implicit memory performance. For instance, if an individual is discouraged from engaging in a meaningful analysis of a stimulus, recall of that stimulus will be impaired, but implicit memory, as exhibited by performance on a word-completion task, will not (Jacoby and Dallas 1981; Schachter and Graf 1986).

More recent studies have found that changes in state, such as those that occur in the presence of clinical depression (Danion et al. 1991) or that are induced by the administration of alcohol (Hashtroudi et al. 1984) or benzodiazepines (Danion et al. 1989; Fang et al. 1987), produce dissociations in which explicit but not implicit memory is impaired.

# Affective and Perceptual-Sensory Aspects of Implicit Memory

Many of the demonstrations of implicit memory, or "knowledge without awareness," show that learning, perceptions, judgments, and actions occurring without conscious awareness are expressed by tasks that strongly emphasize affective reactions to concrete stimuli or motor-perceptual skills, thereby providing substantial evidence that implicit memory has a strong perceptual-sensory component.

## Implicit Perception

The earliest studies demonstrating knowledge without awareness focused on the phenomenon of subliminal perception. In these studies, subjects were presented with stimuli below the range of consciousness, manipulated by means of tachistoscopic or dichotic listening presentations. Despite the absence of conscious awareness of the stimuli, the subjects' behaviors indicated that they had perceived, judged, and interpreted the information presented (see Erdelyi 1985 and Safran and Greenberg 1987 for reviews). In one of the first dichotic listening studies, Corteen and Wood (1972) found that when words that had previously been related to a shock experience were presented to the nonattending channel, subjects would produce skin-conductance changes consistent with registration of a shock event. It was also found that words that bore a semantic relationship to the shock words produced a similar skin response. These findings suggested that emotional/physiological responses to stimuli and related information could occur even when those stimuli were presented outside of conscious awareness.

This line of early dichotic listening research has been severely criticized on methodological grounds concerning whether or not the presented stimuli are indeed out of conscious awareness (Holender 1986). More recent studies using new experimental techniques have more convincingly demonstrated the subliminal character of the stimuli presentation and have produced effects similar to those reported in the earlier studies (Cheeseman and Merikle 1986; Marcel 1983a, 1983b). A variety of studies employing subliminal-perception paradigms have shown the influences of nonconscious processes on affective judgments (Kunst-Wilson and Zajonc 1980; Wilson 1979), evaluative and social judgments (Bargh and Pietromonaco 1982), and shifts in psychopathological states (see Silverman 1983; Weinberger and Hardaway 1991).

## Implicit Recognition

Most of the research concerning implicit and explicit memory has used repetition priming tasks and has contrasted them with conventional tests of explicit memory such as recall and recognition. Unlike conventional memory tests, priming tasks do not involve explicit reference to any information to which the subject has been exposed; nevertheless, performance is influenced by such information. A priming effect is obtained when responses to a stimulus are facilitated as a result of recent exposure to that stimulus; this performance facilitation occurs without the subject's conscious recollection of the previous exposure. For example, in a word-completion task, subjects are asked to complete a three-letter fragment (e.g., suf___) with the first word that comes to mind; a priming effect is obtained when subjects demonstrate a significant preference to complete the fragment so as to form a word recently seen in the experimental setting (e.g., suffuse) rather than a word that has a higher frequency in the language (e.g., suffer) (Danion et al. 1991; Graf et al. 1984; Warrington and Weiskrantz 1982). Other tasks used to assess priming effects are word-fragment completion (Tulving et al. 1982), word identification (Jacoby and Dallas 1981), lexical decision (Scarborough et al. 1979), and reading of a transformed script (Kolers 1975, 1976; Masson 1984).

One interesting aspect of priming effects is that, compared with explicit memory effects, they rely more heavily on the reexperiencing of the specific sensory and perceptual—as opposed to the semantic or meaningful—aspects of the previous exposure. Various lines of evidence are offered in support of this view.

First, priming effects can be obtained with stimuli that have only sensory-perceptual features and no inherent meaning, such as dots and line patterns (Musen and Treisman 1990). Second, priming effects are diminished when the words in the initial exposure phase and the implicit memory phase are mismatched in presentation modality (e.g., visual-auditory) rather than matched (e.g., visual-visual or auditory-auditory); this discrepancy is not demonstrated in explicit memory tasks (see MacLeod and Bassilli 1989; Roediger et al. 1989). In a smaller subset of studies, *no* priming effects were obtained when modalities were mismatched, whereas explicit memory effects were obtained regardless of presentation modality (Graf et al. 1985; Kirsner et al. 1983; Roediger and Blaxton 1987a, 1987b). These data suggest that priming effects are significantly, if not primarily, influenced by the perceptual and sensory characteristics of the stimuli or of the associated processing events.

## Implicit Learning

Researchers have explored the range of potential rules that can be learned and applied without awareness. Lewicki (1986) showed that subjects easily learned covariations between certain stimulus characteristics (e.g., long/short hair) of individuals shown in photographs and particular personality traits (e.g., kind/persistent) given as descriptions of them. Subjects were presented with photographs of individuals who had little in common in their appearance. Descriptions of the individuals as kind or persistent varied across several facial features except that each adjective was consistently matched with a certain hair length. At a later point, subjects were presented with another group of photographs and asked whether the individuals in the photos appeared "kind" or "persistent." Their responses to these questions systematically varied according to whether the person had long or short hair, although the subjects could neither specify the reason for their choice nor relate it to the earlier phase of the experiment. In sum, the subjects learned a rule that related a judgment concerning a personality characteristic with a relatively low-salience physical feature without being aware that they had done so.

## Implicit Judgments

The first assessments of implicit and explicit memory effects on judgments occurred within the context of the subliminal-perception paradigm. In a study by Kunst-Wilson and Zajonc (1980), geometric shapes were subliminally presented to subjects. Explicit memory was evaluated by a forced choice recognition test in which subjects were presented with one new item and one old item. Subjects performed at chance level, which did not provide evidence for their recollection of the previously seen stimuli. Nevertheless, when subjects were asked simply to judge which of an old/new word stimuli pair they liked better, they consistently chose shapes they had seen before, suggesting the presence of implicit memory for the stimuli.

Another line of research indicates that preference judgments for clearly detectable stimuli are governed by rules of which there is no awareness. Nisbett and Wilson (1977), for example, found that when consumers were asked to say which of an array of similar goods (e.g., stockings) was of the highest quality, they tended to choose the rightmost item. Although this effect was quite strong, an in-depth query indicated that the participants had no awareness of that selection criterion and, furthermore, rather vigorously denied using it when it was raised as a possible explanation for their behavior.

## Implicit Behavior

Behavior resulting from implicitly learned and implicitly used motor skills has been ingeniously demonstrated in studies with non-impaired subjects. These studies suggest that motor patterns and their sensory consequences are cognitively represented. Such routines are believed to be accessible to conscious awareness—for example, when an individual is planning an act or evaluating its possible consequences. However, it is clear that these motor routines often influence behavior without conscious awareness.

In an example of this type of research, Van den Bergh et al. (1990) showed typists and nontypists pairs of letters and asked which of two combinations they liked better. One category of letter combinations consisted of letter pairs that would be typed (according to touch-typing rules) with the same finger; the other, of pairs that would be typed with different fingers. Compared with the nontypists, the typists preferred the different-finger letter combinations. These researchers suggested that the typists' preference arose from well-encoded motor rules for touch typing in which different-finger letter combinations allow for cooperative motor actions whereas same-finger letter combinations produce competitive motor responses. Nevertheless, when subjects were shown separate lists of all the same-finger letter combinations and all the different-finger combinations, not a single subject was able to identify the categorical difference between the two sets of letters.

Klatzky et al. (1989, experiment 4) evaluated the extent to which engaging in a motor movement would facilitate sensibility judgments about sentences concerning the movement. Subjects learned and practiced handshapes (e.g., clench, poke) in association with an iconic cue that bore some visual relationship to the motor movement (e.g., clench = > > > >). It was found that subjects' judgment time for phrases such as "clench the newspaper" (versus "clench the window") was facilitated when the motor instruction was preceded by a relevant iconic cue. Presumably, the presentation of the icon primed the memory representation of the motor movement and the associated information about its interaction with objects, thus facilitating judgments about these movements.

Although this study did not investigate the relationship between implicit and explicit memory, the priming effect obtained suggests the presence of implicit memory for the functional aspects of certain sensory-motor patterns.

A further set of observations about implicit memory for sensory-motor routines concerns cases of neurological amnesia. One remarkable characteristic of individuals with this type of amnesia is that despite a striking inability to consciously recall or report any number of experiences, they are still able to perform well on sensory-motor tasks, benefit from practicing sensory-motor skills, and learn new ones. Schachter (1983), for example, described playing a game of golf with an amnesic individual who exhibited extremely poor ability to remember such things as whether he had recently taken a shot and the location of his tee shots (as evidenced by his inability to locate and retrieve the balls). Nonetheless, this individual was able to execute the complex perceptual-motor behaviors required for skillful playing in a fluid and untroubled way.

In summary, a review of the studies described in this section suggests that memory without awareness influences a wide range of cognitive processes and activities: perception, recognition, learning, judgment, and behavior. Furthermore, a growing body of evidence indicates that implicit memory is exhibited primarily in memory about stimuli or processes that involve evaluative-affective or perceptual-motor aspects of experience.

## Selective Aspects of Conscious Memory

Cognitive psychology has a long history in the study of selective attention for both neutral and affective material (see Cloitre 1992 for review). Interestingly, little study or thought has been given to the idea that selective processes operate over memory. In the initial segment of this chapter, I introduced the notion that memory, like attention, may be selective. The following subsections summarize the few studies conducted in this area and discuss their applicability to "motivated forgetting."

## Shifts in Perspective

Anderson and Pichert (1978) showed that initially inaccessible information could be recalled after a shift in perspective. In this study, subjects read a short story about two boys playing hooky from school from the perspective of either a burglar or a person interested in buying a home. After recalling the story once, the subjects were asked to shift perspectives. During the second recall, information emerged that previously had not been recalled. Subjects whose second recall was based on the perspective of the burglar recalled more features of the story (e.g., the presence of jewels in the house) that were relevant to a burglar theme. In contrast, subjects whose second recall was based on the home-buyer theme remembered more details pertinent to that perspective, such as that the house had a leaky roof and a damp basement.

These data show that although a variety of information was initially encoded, instruction—or more broadly, motivation to remember the material in a certain way—guided retrieval to a coherent but selected subset of information. When queried about the absence of information that later emerged, most subjects said that they had simply forgotten the information or that it did not seem relevant despite the request to write down everything they had read. The study shows that individuals remember selectively according to themes or schemas of current interest and that a greater range of information can be elicited with shifts in perspective. This phenomenon is consistent with clinical observations that during therapy, efforts between the therapist and the patient to explore and shift perspective on issues may succeed in eliciting previously inaccessible information.

## Directed Forgetting

Another well-known phenomenon of selective memory is *directed forgetting*. It has been shown that subjects given explicit instructions to forget specific information will on a later memory test indeed show poor memory (both recall and recognition) for the "forget" material (Bjork and Woodward 1973; Horton and Petruk 1980; MacLeod 1975; Wetzel 1975). One common way of obtaining this effect is to present subjects with a series of words and, after each word, indicate that it is to be remembered or forgotten. Generally, the subjects are given an incentive to remember selected words and forget the other words by being told that they will later be tested on the "remember" words and not on the "forget" words. At test, however, subjects are tested on both types of words and show much poorer memory for the "forget" words.

One obvious explanation for this effect is simply that the information the person has been directed to forget has not been as well rehearsed or elaborated during encoding, producing a relatively weak memory trace that is less likely to be successfully retrieved. This explanation has been supported by a few studies (MacLeod 1975; Woodward et al. 1973). However, there is also evidence that when efforts are made to ensure that subjects have satisfactorily encoded test information, later instructions for subjects to forget or remember still produce memory decrements for the "forget" but not the "remember" material.

In a study by Davidson and Bowers (1991), subjects studied to the point of perfect recall a list of 16 words falling into one of four categories (i.e., birds, flowers, alcoholic beverages, furniture). All subjects were then given the suggestion to forget one category of words (the category and all its items were named); half of the subjects received the suggestion under hypnosis and the other half received the suggestion in a normal, alert state. Results indicated that both groups of subjects showed amnesia for the words in the targeted category but not for the nontargeted words.

Some have suggested that the way in which directed forgetting is affected during retrieval processes may be through a global disabling (Davidson and Bowers 1991) or a global inhibition (Bjork 1989; MacLeod 1989) of the retrieval mechanisms. However, the results obtained by Davidson and Bowers (1991) argue against these suggestions. Subjects recalled all categories of information but the targeted set, suggesting that retrieval mechanisms are intact but operating selectively, guided by cues available during retrieval (e.g., retrieve all the birds, all the furniture, and all the flowers, and forget about drinks).

The evidence from the attention research has firmly established that individuals scan the external environment and select out information for further processing. It does not seem unlikely that a search through memory can be similarly selective. Individuals may use certain cues to guide their memory search (cues associated with the "remember" but *not* the "forget" instructions), thereby enhancing retrieval for the "remember" but not the "forget" information. This suggestion is consistent with a line of research that has shown that when cues used during retrieval "match" very specific information of the stored memory (e.g., a word that rhymes with the target word or that identifies the category of word), that information is more likely to be remembered than when a cue is not available or is in some way mismatched (Tulving and Thompson 1973). Thus, for example, if subjects are using cues such as birds or furniture to guide their memory, they are less likely to recall information about drinks. It would not seem unreasonable to assume that affective state or the affective valence of a stimulus might be used as a retrieval cue during a directed memory search. If an individual wishes to avoid recalling a negative or threatening memory, he or she might temporarily generate a positive affective state and use this affective state as a cue during a memory search. The individual would then be more likely to find memories that match the positive affective state and less likely to retrieve a negatively toned memory.

In summary, selective memory processes show flexibility in the range and specificity of stimuli to which they can be applied. Directed forgetting, for example, can occur with individual words (MacLeod 1989; Paller 1990), with a list of words (Bjork 1989), or with a subset of individually presented words that share a common characteristic (Davidson and Bowers 1991). This flexibility is consistent with clinical reports of amnesia for emotionally upsetting events: some patients have no memory for the entirety of an event, whereas others forget only a selected portion.

Directed forgetting may operate in one of two ways: 1) an event may be immediately tagged as an event to forget and thus may never be well encoded, leading to poorer memory; or 2) an event may be well encoded, and poor memory for it might be a result of a mismatch between the information represented in memory and that given in a retrieval cue. Both of these formulations have merit and seem consistent with clinical observations. It is easy to imagine that some experiences (e.g., going through an embarrassing but not significant social encounter) may simply not be well encoded as a result of a self-instruction to forget that occurs almost simultaneously with the event. Alternatively, there may be events that are well processed at the time of their occurrence but for which a person develops, at some later point, a motivation to forget. For example, Freud (1901/1960), in "The Psychopathology of Everyday Life," described a writer who suddenly could not find his pen and papers on an occasion when he would have preferred to be out taking a stroll. A selective memory search in which the writer was scanning his memory for the location of his walking stick rather than his pen might make the retrieval of the pen a low-probability event.

The studies described in this section demonstrate that recall and retrieval of specific information can be significantly impaired under a variety of conditions. These findings contributed to characterizing one aspect of functional amnesia—namely, that by the processes of selective attention (or avoidance) of information in the memory field, certain designated information can be temporarily forgotten. It should be noted, however, that the studies have all been performed in assessment of explicit memory (free or cued recall and recognition) and are silent in regard to the potential selectivity in implicit memory.

## Dissociation of Implicit and Explicit Memory

If it can be successfully argued that the selective memory effects obtained with the directed-forgetting or other paradigms would not be obtained in tests of implicit memory, then a model of functional amnesia would be completely articulated. The final step in establishing the feasibility of the model is to suggest that the types of cognitive manipulations that impair or impede conscious or explicit memory have no effect on implicit memory, leaving the memory for traumatic or other types of events intact and indirectly or implicitly expressed through behaviors, slips of the tongue, or changes in affective states or judgments.

What argument can be made for the dissociation of selective memory processes between implicit and explicit memory? The broad range of types of dissociation obtained between implicit and explicit memory suggests a generalization about the character of this dissociation. Research studies indicate that explicit memory is susceptible to disruption through a variety of agents and manipulations that do not affect implicit memory. Implicit memory remains unperturbed despite the presence of neurological damage, the administration of alcohol or benzodiazepines, or the presence of clinical depression. Some have suggested that explicit memory represents the operation of higher-level but more flexible and fragile cognitive activities—that is, the "executive functions" of the mind—such as goal identification and decision-making processes. Implicit memory, in contrast, may represent a more primitive, long-standing, and enduring form of memory that involves primarily motor and perceptual-sensory activity. Consistent with this view are studies indicating that whereas explicit memory develops and declines over the life span, implicit memory is relatively developed in young children (Naito and Komatsu 1993) and remains intact among the elderly (Howard 1992). Thus, experimental manipulations described earlier in this chapter, such as shifts in perspective and directed forgetting, may be effective in producing impaired recollection of a specific event but leave untouched those "memories" of the experience that represent expressions of the relatively imperturbable implicit memory.

At least one study that used a directed-forgetting paradigm has shown that such a strategy influences explicit memory but has no effect on implicit memory. In this study (Paller 1990), subjects were asked to semantically evaluate a series of words presented in one of two colors. In a counterbalanced design, subjects were told that one color indicated that the word should be forgotten, and the other color, that the word should be remembered. Subjects' performance on two explicit memory tasks was influenced by the forgetting instruction, with poorer performance on the "forget" words; in contrast, implicit memory was equivalent for the "forget" and the "remember" words.

In Paller's study, the motivation to remember or forget a particular word derived from the subject's desire or willingness to follow the experimenter's instructions. This type of strategy, however, might also be applied under conditions in which the motivation to forget is prompted by a desire to avoid painful or negative memories. An individual may be motivated to forget an upsetting event, such as overhearing something negative said about him. If this individual were to engage in a process such as directed forgetting, we might expect that the exercise would succeed in minimizing conscious recollection of the episode but would not exert any influence on the expressions of implicit memory. When presented with any salient stimulus that represents characteristics of the forgotten event, such as the voice of the person who spoke ill of him, the individual might experience a feeling of distress or discomfort without understanding its source.

To evaluate this possibility, future studies should investigate the contributions of personality and of the emotional characteristics of the presented information to the memory performance observed in directed-forgetting or other types of paradigms. Individuals predisposed to avoid the processing of painful information may be more skilled than others at following instructions to remember some things (e.g., pleasant) but forget others (e.g., unpleasant).

My colleagues and I recently compared directed-forgetting skills in individuals with a history of childhood sexual abuse with those skills in individuals without a history of abuse, and have found that although the groups do not differ in their performance on an implicit memory task for a series of words to which they were exposed, the sexually abused group tended to demonstrate greater directed-forgetting skills (Cloitre et al. 1996). It has been suggested that individuals sexually abused as children develop skill in avoiding or ignoring information—or, alternatively, attend to positive or neutral (i.e., nontraumatizing) information—in order to maximize survival in a situation from which they cannot escape (Freyd 1996; Terr 1994). This is one example of the type of research that can be conducted to test a model of motivated cognitive processing. Such research might also yield an improved understanding of the cognitive-affective processing style of a population about which little is known.

# Recovery of Lost Traumatic Memories

In most of this chapter, I have focused on developing a cognitive model that can explain and test the phenomenon of functional amnesia. The model is intended to account for amnesia for a variety of events, including the trauma of childhood abuse. Given the current political climate concerning the veracity of memories of childhood abuse, some discussion is warranted concerning the quantity and nature of child abuse memories and cognitive science perspectives on them, including discussion of how once "forgotten" memories may be recovered.

## The Adaptive Function of Amnesia for Childhood Abuse Memories

The general argument stated earlier—that selectivity of memory operates in the service of adaptation to the environment—is applicable to memories of childhood abuse. Traumatic memories of childhood abuse, especially of abuse by caretaking figures, may be "forgotten" so as to maximize functioning in daily life.

The parent-child relationship is one in which the child is enormously dependent on the parent for basic care such as safety and nurturance. The child who is sexually and/or physically abused by a caretaker has limited resources with which to avoid the abuse or find alternative sources of care. Thus, he or she may rely on psychological resources such as temporarily "forgetting" or putting away memories of the parent as abuser in order to maximally relate to the parent as a source of care.

Lost memories may be recovered when such "forgetting" is no longer needed. This seems to occur when the traumatic memory becomes significantly less threatening, such as when an individual from an abusive family leaves home. In addition, recollection of abuse may occur when the amnesia becomes maladaptive, as it is often does outside the abusive environment, and the individual begins to search for the source of his or her difficulties in functioning or unexplained symptomatology, such as chronic depression or panic attacks.

## The Frequency of Amnesia for Childhood Abuse

A few studies have attempted to assess the prevalence of amnesia for childhood abuse. The best study available to date (L. M. Williams 1994) concerns the recollection of abuse among 100 women for whom documentation of childhood abuse existed in the form of hospital records and medical case histories. All of the women had been brought before the age of 12 to a city-hospital emergency department for treatment of sexual and/or physical abuse and collection of forensic evidence. When the women were interviewed as adults (ages 18 to 31 years) about a variety of life events and experiences, including sexual abuse, 38% either did not recall or chose not to report the abuse. Two important points emerge from this study. First, the majority of the women recalled and reported their abuse, indicating that abused women provide veridical and accurate information about their abuse histories. Second, the existence of independent documentation of the abuse enabled a reliable assessment of "false negative" responses (i.e., failure to report or to recall abuse that occurred). Thus, although the extent to which women report false memories is unknown, we are now certain that a substantial minority of women either do not recall or deny experiencing abuse that has occurred. Accordingly, attention should be given to this problem.

Two studies that surveyed individuals receiving abuse-related psychotherapy found that between 64% (Herman and Schatzow 1987) and 59.3% (Briere and Conte 1993) of the patients reported either partial or full amnesia for their abuse experiences. In contrast, a recent study by Loftus et al. (1994) found that of 52 women in treatment for substance abuse, only 31% reported partial or complete amnesia for sexual abuse that occurred during some period in their lives.

Thus, the rates of reported amnesia range from moderate (31%, 38%) to high (59%, 64%), with the latter rates appearing in abuse-related psychotherapy samples. It is difficult to know what to make of this discrepancy. It may be that the psychotherapy patients underwent more severe abuse and accordingly experienced greater posttraumatic sequelae, including amnesia for the experience. In the course of therapy, these memories may emerge if the therapeutic context is experienced by the patients as sufficiently nonthreatening and supportive. An alternative view recently discussed in scientific journals (Loftus 1993) is that overzealous therapists implant or suggest "false memories" in the patient's mind—that is, for any number of reasons, a therapist suggests to a patient that he or she might have been abused, thereby initiating an avenue of discussion in which the patient may not have otherwise engaged. This issue, currently highly politicized, deserves systematic scientific investigation. From a cognitive science perspective, both the emergence of lost memories and the confabulation or creation of false memories are possible. Laboratory studies consistent with these two phenomena are briefly discussed below.

## Cognitive Mechanisms to Explain Abuse Memory Phenomena

### Hypermnesia

Recovery of memories of abuse during sustained discussion such as that which may occur in psychotherapy may be legitimate and may represent an example of the well-documented phenomenon of hypermnesia (see Erdelyi 1985 for review). It is well known from laboratory studies and the experience of daily life that recall of specific information diminishes with time (i.e., the Ebbinghaus forgetting curve). However, a reverse effect known as *hypermnesia* has been identified wherein recall, rather than deteriorating, improves with time and effort. Although various interpretations for this effect have been offered, it has recently been explained in terms of the implicit/explicit memory distinction—or, more broadly, in terms of contrasting notions of accessible versus available memory (Kihlstrom and Barnhardt 1993). Hypermnesia may reflect the retrieval of information that had previously been available in memory (implicit memory) but not accessible to conscious retrieval. The mechanisms by which memories become more accessible remain to be specified. However, some artifactual explanations have been ruled out (e.g., shifts in reporting criteria), and some aspects of hypermnesia have been reliably established.

Overall, the studies of hypermnesia suggest that active and effortful review of associated information may facilitate increases in the accessibility of "lost" memories. Interestingly, the laboratory studies have assessed the influence of several types of "cognitive effort"—for example, free associating, fantasizing, and just plain "thinking"—on hypermnesia and have found that they all produce the effect. These results suggest that a variety of cognitive processes can cause hypermnesia and, hence, that various treatment approaches employing different cognitive strategies—for example, the free association of psychoanalysis and the focused and conscious effort of cognitive therapy—can produce hypermnesia or recovery of lost memories.

Of additional interest is the observation that the hypermnesic effect occurs more readily when imaginal rather than verbal processing of material is required (Erdelyi and Becker 1974). This observation is relevant to the recovery of traumatic memories, given that such memories appear to be strongly encoded in a perceptual-sensory form, as exhibited in flashbacks, nightmares, and unexpected visceral sensations. It is often the case that psychotherapy focusing on the processing of traumatic memories initially makes use of these consciously available aspects of the traumatic event and works toward the recovery of a fuller memory. Thus, the hypermnesic effect may be inadvertently enhanced in trauma therapy because the initial memory with which treatment work begins will most likely be an image or some other type of perceptual-sensory memory.

## Alterations of Recollection

An alternative interpretation of the putative recovery of abuse memories is that such memories are distortions or alterations of innocuous past events. These distortions may be the result of exposure to misleading information, such as mistaken assumptions or inadvertent suggestions on the part of the therapist or inaccurate inferences on the part of the patient of a history of abuse based on the presence of symptomatology that has been reported in the self-help or scientific literature to be highly associated with childhood abuse. Under this scenario, the longer the individual considers and reworks his or her history to assess the possibility of early abuse, the more potential exists for distortion to occur.

Consistent with this line of thought is a series of laboratory studies documenting "malleability of memory" (Loftus and Christianson 1989). Loftus and colleagues developed a "postevent misinformation" paradigm with which to systematically study the extent to which and the conditions under which memory can be distorted. It has been found that if subjects are provided with false information in a subtle way, often in the guise of a question concerning an event they have witnessed in a series of slides, subjects will often assimilate this information into their story narrative and report the information as "true" during later questioning.

Consider a typical example of the paradigm. A subject is shown a series of slides in which a red Datsun is driving along a side street toward an intersection containing a stop sign. The series of slides concludes with the Datsun making a right turn and knocking down a pedestrian at the crosswalk. The subject is later fed misinformation in the form of a question: "Did another car pass the red Datsun while it was stopped at the yield sign?" In the final phase of the study, subjects are shown slides that match either the original slide with the stop sign or the misinformation they received via the question (i.e., a slide with a yield sign). Loftus et al. (1978) found that in a yes/no recognition task of the target slides, the subjects' hit rate (true positives) was 71%, whereas their false-alarm rate (false positives) was 70%. As Loftus and colleagues have noted, these data indicate that subjects have no ability to discriminate between the sign they saw and the sign they did not see.

Although these data suggest that reports of events can be manipulated, perhaps a more interesting question concerns the "fate" of the original memory. One possibility is that the original memory has been altered and thus no longer exists (Loftus and Christianson 1989). Alternatively, it is possible that the original memory is still encoded in memory but is less accessible due to the introduction of the postevent information. This issue remains unresolved. Furthermore, there is no principled reason to dismiss the idea that both processes may operate, depending on the event, the person, and the context in which the memory is to be retrieved.

Parallel questions can be raised concerning memories for real-life trauma. Can memories of childhood events be transformed into sexual or other types of trauma as a result of postevent information (e.g., a therapist's suggestion)? Do original memories continue to exist despite the presence of altered formulations? These questions can be framed more specifically within the implicit/explicit memory framework. For example, memory tasks such as the recognition test used in the Loftus et al. studies reveal the manipulation or transformation only of explicit memory. It remains to be seen whether tests of implicit memory would show similar transformations following exposure to misinformation.

## Chapter Summary

The primary goal of this chapter was to present a model of functional amnesia within the context of the implicit/explicit memory distinction. Four requirements to be met by this framework in order for it to be considered a model of functional amnesia with sufficient explanatory power were specified. Several studies were presented and reviewed in connection with each of the four requirements. Support for this model was deemed sufficient to warrant further investigation. The application of tasks such as the directed-forgetting paradigm to abused or other clinical populations with histories of memory disturbance (e.g., posttraumatic stress disorder [PTSD] patients) may help elucidate the processes or character of memory disturbances beyond what we can know on the basis of clinical observation. The discussion of the research related to the recovery of abuse memories identified ways in which studies of human cognition can help ground discussion of abuse memories in a scientific context. In this discussion, the implicit/explicit memory distinction was presented as useful both in interpreting current studies and in indicating directions for future research. It should also be noted that clinical phenomena such as functional amnesia, dissociation, and dissociative identity disorder present a challenge to theories of cognitive science, identifying the need for more sophisticated and inclusive models of affective-cognitive functioning. In summary, the emerging collaboration between cognitive science and psychiatry shows promise of producing a cross-fertilization of ideas and observations that will enhance both theories of mind and treatment of individuals who suffer from mental disorders.

# References

Anderson RC, Pichert JW: Recall of previously unrecallable information following a shift in perspective. Journal of Verbal Learning and Verbal Behavior 17:1–12, 1978

Bargh JA, Pietromonaco P: Automatic information processing and social perception: the influence of trait information presented outside of conscious awareness on impression formation. J Pers Soc Psychol 43:437–449, 1982

Bjork RA: Retrieval inhibition as an adaptive mechanism in human memory, in Varieties of Memory and Consciousness: Essays in Honour of Endel Tulving. Edited by Roediger HL, Craik FIM. Hillsdale, NJ, Lawrence Erlbaum, 1989, pp 309–330

Bjork RA, Woodward AE Jr: Directed forgetting of individual words in free recall. J Exp Psychol 99:22–27, 1973

Bowers KS: On being unconsciously influenced and informed, in The Unconscious Reconsidered. Edited by Bowers KS, Meichenbaum D. New York, Wiley, 1984, pp 227–272

Breuer J, Freud S: On the psychical mechanism of hysterical phenomena: preliminary communication (1893), in The Standard Edition of the Complete Psychological Works of Sigmund Freud, Vol 2. Translated and edited by Strachey J. London, Hogarth Press, 1955, pp 1–18

Briere J, Conte J: Self-reported amnesia for abuse in adults molested as children. Journal of Traumatic Stress 6:21–31, 1993

Cheeseman J, Merikle PM: Word recognition and consciousness, in Reading Research: Advances in Theory and Practice, Vol 5. Edited by Besner D, Waller TG, Mackinnon GE. New York, Academic Press, 1986, pp 311–352

Claparède E: Recognition and "me-ness" (1911), in Organization and Pathology of Thought. Edited by Rapaport D. New York, Columbia University Press, 1951, pp 58–75

Cloitre M: Avoidance of emotional processing: a cognitive science perspective, in Cognitive Science and Clinical Disorders. Edited by Stein DJ, Young JE. San Diego, CA, Academic Press, 1992, pp 19–44

Cloitre M, Cancienne J, Brodsky B, et al: Memory performance among women with parental abuse histories: enhanced directed forgetting or directed remembering? J Abnorm Psychol 105:204–211, 1996

Corteen RS, Wood B: Autonomic responses to shock associated threat words. J Exp Psychol 94:308–313, 1972

Danion JM, Zimmermann MA, Willard-Schroeder D, et al: Diazepam induces a dissociation between explicit and implicit memory. Psychopharmacology 99:238–243, 1989

Danion JM, Willard-Schroeder D, Zimmermann MA, et al: Explicit memory and repetition priming in depression. Arch Gen Psychiatry 48:707–711, 1991

Davidson TM, Bowers KS: Selective hypnotic amnesia: is it a successful attempt to forget or an unsuccessful attempt to remember? J Abnorm Psychol 100:133–143, 1991

Ellenberger HF: The Discovery of the Unconscious: The History and Evolution of Dynamic Psychiatry. New York, Basic Books, 1970

Erdelyi MH: Psychoanalysis: Freud's Cognitive Psychology. New York, WH Freeman, 1985

Erdelyi MH, Becker J: Hypermnesia for pictures: incremental memory for pictures not for words in multiple recall trials. Cognitive Psychology 6:159–171, 1974

Erdelyi MH, Goldberg B: Let's not sweep repression under the rug: toward a cognitive psychology of repression, in Functional Disorders of Memory. Edited by Kihlstrom JF, Evans FJ. Hillsdale, NJ, Lawrence Erlbaum, 1979, pp 355–402

Fang JC, Hinrichs JV, Ghoneim MM: Diazepam and memory: evidence for spared memory function. Pharmacol Biochem Behav 28:347–352, 1987

Freyd JJ: Betrayal Trauma Theory: The Logic of Forgetting Abuse. Cambridge, MA, Harvard University Press, 1996

Freud S: The neuro-psychoses of defense (1894), in The Standard Edition of the Complete Psychological Works of Sigmund Freud, Vol 3. Translated and edited by Strachey J. London, Hogarth Press, 1962, pp 41–68

Freud S: The psychopathology of everyday life (1901), in The Standard Edition of the Complete Psychological Works of Sigmund Freud, Vol 6. Translated and edited by Strachey J. London, Hogarth Press, 1960

Graf P, Squire LR, Mandler G: The information that amnesic patients do not forget. J Exp Psychol Learn Mem Cogn 10:164–178, 1984

Graf P, Shimamura AP, Squire LR: Priming across modalities and priming across category levels: extending the domain of preserved function in amnesia. J Exp Psychol Learn Mem Cogn 11:385–395, 1985

Hashtroudi S, Parker ES, Delisi LE, et al: Intact retention in acute alcohol amnesia. J Exp Psychol Learn Mem Cogn 10:156–163, 1984

Herman JL, Schatzow E: Recovery and verification of memories of childhood sexual trauma. Psychoanalytic Psychology 4:1–14, 1987

Holender D: Semantic activation without conscious identification in dichotic listening, parafoveal vision, and visual masking: a survey and appraisal. Behavioral and Brain Sciences 9:1–66, 1986

Holmes DS: Investigations of repression: differential recall of material experimentally or naturally associated with ego threat. Psychol Bull 81:632–653, 1974

Horton KD, Petruk R: Set differentiation and depth of processing in the directed forgetting paradigm. J Exp Psychol Hum Learn 6:599–610, 1980

Howard DV: Implicit memory: an expanding picture of cognitive aging (Schaie KW, Series Editor). Annual Review of Gerontology and Geriatrics 11:1–22, 1992

Jacoby LL, Dallas M: On the relationship between autobiographical memory and perceptual learning. J Exp Psychol Gen 110:306–340, 1981

Janet P: L'amnésie continué [Continuous amnesia]. Revue Generale Des Sciences 4:167–179, 1893

Johnson MK, Kim JK, Risse G: Do alcoholic Korsakoff's syndrome patients acquire affective reactions? J Exp Psychol Learn Mem Cogn 11:27–36, 1985

Kihlstrom JF: The cognitive unconscious. Science 237:1445–1452, 1987

Kihlstrom JF, Barnhardt TM: The self-regulation of memory: for better or worse, with and without hypnosis, in Handbook of Mental Control. Edited by Wegner DM, Pennebaker JW. Englewood Cliffs, NJ, Prentice Hall, 1993, pp 88–125

Kirsner K, Milech D, Standen P: Common and modality-specific processes in the mental lexicon. Memory and Cognition 11:621–630, 1983

Klatzky RL, Pellegrino JW, McCloskey BP, et al: Can you squeeze a tomato? the role of motor representations in semantic sensibility judgments. Journal of Memory and Language 28:56–77, 1989

Kolers PA: Memorial consequences of automatized encoding. J Exp Psychol Hum Learn 1:689–701, 1975

Kolers PA: Reading a year later. J Exp Psychol Human Learning and Memory 2:554–565, 1976

Kunst-Wilson WR, Zajonc RB: Affective discrimination of stimuli that cannot be recognized. Science 207:557–558, 1980

Lewicki P: Processing information about covariations that cannot be articulated. J Exp Psychol Learn Mem Cogn 12:135–146, 1986

Loftus E: The reality of repressed memories. Am Psychol 48:518–537, 1993

Loftus E, Christianson SA: Malleability of memory for emotional events, in Aversion, Avoidance and Anxiety. Edited by Archer T, Nilsson LG. New York, Lawrence Erlbaum, 1989, pp 311–322

Loftus E, Miller DG, Burns HJ: Semantic integration of verbal information into a visual memory. J Exp Psychol Hum Learn 4:19–31, 1978

Loftus E, Polonsky S, Fullilove M: Memories of childhood abuse: remembering and repressing. Psychology of Women Quarterly 18:67–84, 1994

MacLeod CM: Long-term recognition and recall following directed forgetting. Journal of Exp Psychol Hum Learn 1:271–279, 1975

MacLeod CM: Directed forgetting affects both direct and indirect tests of memory. J Exp Psychol Learn Mem Cogn 15:13–21, 1989

MacLeod CM, Bassili JN: Are implicit and explicit tests differentially sensitive to item-specific vs. relational information? in Implicit Memory: Theoretical Issues. Edited by Lewandowsky S, Dunn J, Kirsner K. Hillsdale, NJ, Lawrence Erlbaum, 1989, pp 159–173

Marcel AJ: Conscious and unconscious perception: experiments on visual masking and word recognition. Cognitive Psychology 15:197–237, 1983a

Marcel AJ: Conscious and unconscious perception: an approach to the relations between phenomenal experience and perceptual processes. Cognitive Psychology 15:238–300, 1983b

Masson MEJ: Memory for the surface structure of sentences: remembering with and without awareness. Journal of Verbal Learning and Verbal Behavior 23:579–592, 1984

Musen G, Treisman A: Implicit and explicit memory for visual patterns. J Exp Psychol Learn Mem Cogn 16:127–137, 1990

Naito M, Komatsu S: Processes involved in childhood development of implicit memory, in Implicit Memory: New Directions in Cognition, Development and Neurology. Edited by Graf P, Masson MJ. Hillsdale, NJ, Lawrence Erlbaum, 1993

Nisbett RE, Wilson TD: Telling more than we can know: verbal reports on mental processes. Psychol Rev 84:231–259, 1977

Paller KA: Recall and stem-completion priming have different electrophysiological correlates and are modified differentially by directed forgetting. J Exp Psychol Learn Mem Cogn 16:1021–1032, 1990

Perry C, Lawrence JR: Mental processes outside awareness: the contributions of Freud and Janet, in The Unconscious Reconsidered. Edited by Bowers KS, Meichenbaum D. New York, Wiley, 1984, pp 9–48

Richardson-Klavehn A, Bjork RA: Measures of memory. Annu Rev Psychol 39:475–543, 1988

Roediger HL, Blaxton TA: Effects of varying modality, surface features, and retention interval on priming in word fragment completion. Memory and Cognition 15:379–388, 1987a

Roediger HL, Blaxton TA: Retrieval modes produce dissociations in memory for surface information, in Memory and Cognitive Processes: The Effinghaus Centennial Conference. Edited by Gorfein D, Hoffman RR. Hillsdale, NJ, Lawrence Erlbaum, 1987b, pp 349–377

Roediger HL, Weldon MS, Challis BH: Explaining dissociations between implicit and explicit measures of retention: a processing account, in Varieties of Memory and Consciousness: Essays in Honour of Endel Tulving. Edited by Roediger HL, Craik FIM. Hillsdale, NJ, Lawrence Erlbaum, 1989, pp 3–41

Safran JD, Greenberg LS: Affect and the unconscious: a cognitive perspective, in Theories of the Unconscious and Theories of the Self. Edited by Stern R. Hillsdale, NJ, Lawrence Erlbaum, 1987, pp 191–212

Scarborough DL, Gerard L, Cortese C: Accessing lexical memory: the transfer of word repetition effects across task and modality. Memory and Cognition 7:3–12, 1979

Schachter DL: Amnesia observed: remembering and forgetting in a natural environment. J Abnorm Psychol 92:236–242, 1983

Schachter DL: Implicit memory: history and current status. J Exp Psychol Learn Mem Cogn 13:501–518, 1987

Schachter DL, Graf P: Effects of elaborative processing on implicit and explicit memory for new associations. J Exp Psychol Learn Mem Cogn 12:432–444, 1986

Silverman LH: The subliminal psychodynamic activation method: overview and comprehensive listing of studies, in Empirical Studies of Psychoanalytic Theories, Vol 1. Edited by Masling J. Hillsdale, NJ, Lawrence Erlbaum, 1983

Tobias BA, Kihlstrom JF, Schachter DL: Emotion and Implicit Memory, in The Handbook of Emotion and Memory: Research and Theory. Edited by Christianson SA. Hillsdale, NJ, Lawrence Erlbaum, 1992, pp 67–92

Terr L: Unchained Memories: True Stories of Traumatic Memories Lost and Found. New York, Basic Books, 1994

Tulving E, Thompson DM: Encoding specificity and retrieval processes in episodic memory. Psychol Rev 80:352–373, 1973

Tulving E, Schachter DL, Stark HA: Priming effects in word-fragment completion are independent of recognition memory. J Exp Psychol Learn Mem Cogn 8:336–342, 1982

Van den Bergh O, Vrana S, Eelen P: Letters from the heart: affective categorization of letter combinations in typists and nontypists. J Exp Psychol Learn Mem Cogn 16:1153–1161, 1990

Warrington EK, Weiskrantz L: Amnesia: a disconnection syndrome? Neuropsychologia 20:233–248, 1982

Weinberger J, Hardaway R: Separating science from myth in subliminal psychodynamic activation. Clinical Psychology Review 10:727–756, 1991

Wetzel CD: Effect of orienting tasks and cue timing on the free recall of remember- and forget-cued words. J Exp Psychol Hum Learn 1:556–566, 1975

Williams JMG, Watts FN, MacLeod CM, et al: Cognitive Psychology and Emotional Disorders. Chichester, UK, Wiley, 1988

Williams LM: Recall of childhood trauma: a prospective study of women's memories of childhood sexual abuse. J Consult Clin Psychol 62:1167–1176, 1994

Wilson WR: Feeling more than we can know: exposure effects without learning. J Pers Soc Psychol 37:811–821, 1979

Woodward AE Jr, Bjork RA, Jongeward RH: Recall and recognition as a function of primary rehearsal. Journal of Verbal Learning and Verbal Behavior 12:608–617, 1973

# Chapter 4

# *How Unconscious Metaphorical Thought Shapes Dreams*

George Lakoff, Ph.D.

## Unconscious Thought in Cognitive Science

Cognitive science brings together empirical techniques for studying the mind from cognitive and developmental psychology, neuroscience, linguistics, and anthropology, as well as the modeling techniques from computer science. The result is an interdisciplinary study of the mind that asks very different questions than psychotherapists ask, and not surprisingly, gets very different answers.

Perhaps the most striking result obtained across the various branches of cognitive science is that most thought is unconscious—though not in the sense that Freud meant by the term. To Freud, unconscious thought was thought that could, in principle, be brought to consciousness. It was thought that was, to a large extent, repressed—too painful to be brought to consciousness. The cognitive unconscious is not like this at all. The kind of unconscious thinking studied by cognitive science cannot be done consciously. It is thinking that is extremely fast, automatic, effortless—and completely normal. It is what we call "common sense"—the most mundane kind of thought.

Moreover, cognitive science tends to study common modes of thought, not the thought of a particular individual or class. Since it studies normal thought processes, it is not concerned with pathology; rather, it is concerned with what is common about how normal people ordinarily make sense of the world. For this reason, cognitive science and psychotherapy have seen themselves as

89

concerned with disjoint subject matter and have barely had any interaction at all.

I think this is unfortunate. To understand psychopathology, one needs to understand the workings of the normal mind. Correspondingly, psychopathology provides challenges to those who study the normal mind. The cognitive unconscious is not at all at odds with the Freudian unconscious. Both exist. But cognitive science has so far had nothing to say about the Freudian unconscious, since the techniques of analysis in the two fields are so different.

At first glance, the Freudian and cognitive forms of the unconscious look very different. For Freud, unconscious thought could be made conscious; but because it is "highly charged," it is repressed. The cognitive unconscious is of a different character. It is part of the mechanism of thought, by nature automatic and typically not subject to conscious control. It need not be highly charged at all; it consists of the most commonplace aspects of our conceptual system.

There are, however, similarities between the Freudian and the cognitive unconscious. What Freud called *symbolization, displacement, condensation,* and *reversal* appear to be the same mechanisms that cognitive scientists refer to as *conceptual metaphor, conceptual metonymy, conceptual blending,* and *irony.* But whereas Freud saw these mechanisms as irrational modes of primary-process thinking, cognitive scientists have found these modes to be an indispensable part of ordinary, rational thought, which is largely unconscious.

The relationship between thought and affect is a recurring theme in cognitive science. Antonio Damasio (1994) has argued that ordinary means–end rationality requires emotional involvement. The argument is based on patients with a form of brain damage that leaves them emotionless; invariably such patients have trouble achieving their goals and make a mess of their lives. Conversely, Zoltàn Kövecses and I have shown that there is a metaphorical logic of emotion concepts (Lakoff 1987, case study 3; Kövecses 1990). Anger, for example, is conceptualized metaphorically in terms of heat, madness, a wild animal, and so on.

This chapter does not in any way attempt to provide an account of any aspect of psychopathology. Nor does it attempt to give a full theory of dreams, nor even to explain what the function of dreams is. Nonetheless, in the cases that happen to have been studied, the dreams all seem to express a deeply important wish, fear, or regret—typically one that the dreamer would not be able to discuss in public. Yet I feel that I have not done enough research on dreams to claim that all dreams work like this. But certainly many do.

The cases discussed all bear on the lives of the dreamers, and all of the dreams, in one way or another, express immediate difficulties in the dreamer's life. This expression of difficulties (and, in some cases, resolutions) is done through the use of our system of conventional metaphors. As we shall see, the system of metaphorical thought that we use in everyday life provides us with a language of dreams.

## Metaphorical Thought

It was discovered in the late 1970s that the mind contains an enormous system of general conceptual metaphors—ways of understanding relatively abstract concepts in terms of those that are more concrete. Much of our everyday language and thought makes use of such conceptual metaphors. To take a simple example, consider the sentence "I'm weighed down by responsibilities." There is a form of metaphorical thought operating here, namely, DIFFICULTIES ARE BURDENS. This way of conceptualizing difficulties can be expressed in many different linguistic forms (e.g., "I'm **carrying a heavy load**," "He's **shouldering** a lot of responsibility," "Get **off my back!**"). As any therapist will immediately recognize, such metaphors can be made real—for example, in posture. Someone weighed down by responsibilities may carry himself as if he had a heavy load on his shoulders. Thus, metaphorical thought does not merely govern language and reasoning but may also be realized in behavior.

This chapter is about the way our ordinary, conventional system of metaphorical thought shapes dreams—and hence may provide a therapist with insights as to the nature of dreams. But before I turn to the discussion of dreams, I should spend a bit of time explicating in detail what I mean by "metaphorical thought."

Imagine a love relationship described as follows:

Our relationship has **hit a dead-end street.**

Here, love is being conceptualized as a journey, with the implication that the relationship is stalled, that the lovers cannot keep going the way they've been going, that they must turn back, or abandon the relationship altogether. This is not an isolated case. English has many everyday expressions that are based on a conceptualization of love as a journey, and they are used not just for talking about love, but for reasoning about it as well. Some are necessarily about love; others can be understood that way:

Look how **far** we've **come.** It's been a **long, bumpy road.** We can't **turn back** now. We're at a **crossroads.** We may have to **go our separate ways.** The relationship isn't **going anywhere.** We're **spinning our wheels.** Our relationship is **off track.** The marriage is **on the rocks.** We may have to **bail out** of this relationship.

These are ordinary, everyday English expressions. They are not poetic, nor are they necessarily used for special rhetorical effect. Those like "Look how far we've come," which aren't necessarily about love, can readily be understood as being about love.

As a linguist and a cognitive scientist, I ask two commonplace questions:

- Is there a general principle governing how these linguistic expressions about journeys are used to characterize love?
- Is there a general principle governing how our patterns of inference about journeys are used to reason about love when expressions such as these are used?

The answer to both is yes. Indeed, there is a single general principle that answers both questions. But it is a general principle that is part of neither the grammar of English nor the English lexicon. Rather, it is part of the conceptual system underlying English: It is a principle for understanding the domain of love in terms of the domain of journeys. The principle can be stated informally as a metaphorical scenario:

> The lovers are travelers on a journey together, with their common life goals seen as destinations to be reached. The relationship is their vehicle, and it allows them to pursue those common goals together. The relationship is seen as fulfilling its purpose as long as it allows them to make progress toward their common goals. The journey isn't easy. There are impediments, and there are places (crossroads) where a decision has to be made about which direction to take and whether to keep traveling together.

The metaphor involves understanding one domain of experience, love, in terms of a very different domain of experience, journeys. More technically, the metaphor can be understood as a mapping (in the mathematical sense) from a source domain (in this case, journeys) to a target domain (in this case, love). The mapping is tightly structured. There are ontological correspondences, according to which entities in the domain of love (the lovers, their common goals, their difficulties, the love relationship, etc.) correspond systematically to entities in the domain of a journey (the travelers, the vehicle, destinations, etc.). To make it easier to remember what mappings exist in the conceptual system, Johnson and I (Lakoff and Johnson 1980) adopted a strategy for naming such mappings by using mnemonics that suggest the mapping. Mnemonic names typically have the form

X is Y,

where X is the name of the target domain and Y is the name of the source domain. In this case, the name of the mapping is LOVE IS A JOURNEY.

When I speak of the LOVE IS A JOURNEY metaphor, I am using a mnemonic for a set of ontological correspondences that characterize a mapping, namely:

### The LOVE IS A JOURNEY Mapping

- The lovers correspond to travelers.
- The love relationship corresponds to the vehicle.
- The lovers' common goals correspond to their common destinations for the journey.
- Difficulties in the relationship correspond to impediments to travel.

It is a common mistake to confuse the name of the mapping, LOVE IS A JOURNEY, for the mapping itself. The mapping is the set of correspondences. Thus, whenever I refer to a metaphor by a mnemonic like LOVE IS A JOURNEY, I will be referring to such a set of correspondences.

The LOVE IS A JOURNEY mapping is a set of ontological correspondences that map knowledge about journeys onto knowledge about love. Such correspondences permit us to reason about love using the knowledge we use to reason about journeys. Let us take an example. Consider the expression, "We're stuck," said by one lover to another about their relationship. How is this expression about travel to be understood as being about their relationship?

"We're stuck" can be used of travel, and when it is, it evokes knowledge about travel. The exact knowledge may vary from person to person, but here is a typical example of the kind of knowledge evoked. The capitalized expressions represent entities in the ontology of travel, that is, in the source domain of the LOVE IS A JOURNEY mapping given above.

Two TRAVELERS are in a VEHICLE, traveling WITH COMMON DESTINATIONS. The VEHICLE encounters some IMPEDIMENT and gets stuck, that is, becomes nonfunctional. If they do nothing, they will not REACH THEIR DESTINATIONS. There are a limited number of alternatives for action:

- They can try to get the VEHICLE moving again, either by fixing it or by getting it past the IMPEDIMENT that stopped it.
- They can remain in the nonfunctional VEHICLE and give up on REACHING THEIR DESTINATIONS.
- They can abandon the VEHICLE.

The alternative of remaining in the nonfunctional VEHICLE takes the least effort but does not satisfy the desire to REACH THEIR DESTINATIONS.

The ontological correspondences that constitute the LOVE IS A JOURNEY metaphor map the ontology of travel onto the ontology of love. In so doing, they map this scenario about travel onto a corresponding love scenario in which the corresponding alternatives for action are seen. Here is the corresponding love scenario that results from applying the correspondences to this knowledge structure. The target-domain entities that are mapped by the correspondences are capitalized:

Two LOVERS are in a LOVE RELATIONSHIP, PURSUING COMMON LIFE GOALS. The RELATIONSHIP encounters some DIFFICULTY, which makes it nonfunctional. If they do nothing, they will not be able to ACHIEVE THEIR LIFE GOALS. There are a limited number of alternatives for action:

- They can try to get the RELATIONSHIP moving again, either by fixing it or by getting it past the DIFFICULTY.
- They can remain in the nonfunctional RELATIONSHIP and give up on ACHIEVING THEIR LIFE GOALS.
- They can abandon the RELATIONSHIP.

The alternative of remaining in the nonfunctional RELATIONSHIP takes the least effort but does not satisfy the desire to ACHIEVE LIFE GOALS.

This is an example of an inference pattern that is mapped from one domain to another. It is via such mappings that we apply knowledge about travel to love relationships.

## Metaphors Are Not Mere Words

What constitutes the LOVE IS A JOURNEY metaphor is not any particular word or expression; it is the ontological mapping across conceptual domains, from the source domain of journeys to the target domain of love. The metaphor is a matter not just of language but also of thought and reason. The language is secondary. The mapping is primary, in that it sanctions the use of source-domain language and inference patterns for target-domain concepts. The mapping is conventional, that is, it is a fixed part of our conceptual system, one of our conventional ways of conceptualizing love relationships.

This view of metaphor is thoroughly at odds with the traditional view of metaphor. The traditional view includes the following claims:

1. Metaphors are linguistic expressions (as opposed to conceptual mappings).
2. Metaphors use words from one literal domain to express concepts in another literal domain, but there is no such thing as metaphorical thought or metaphorical reasoning in which inference patterns from one domain are applied to another domain.
3. Metaphors are based on similarity: words from one domain express similar concepts in other domains.
4. Metaphorical language is not part of ordinary, everyday, conventional language, but rather of poetic or especially rhetorical language.

All of these claims are false. For example, if metaphors were merely linguistic expressions, we would expect different linguistic expressions to be different metaphors. Thus, "We've hit a dead-end street" would constitute one metaphor. "We can't turn back now" would constitute another, entirely different metaphor. "Their marriage is on the rocks" would involve still a different metaphor. And so on, for dozens of examples. Yet we don't seem to have dozens of different metaphors here. We have one metaphor, in which love is conceptualized as a journey. The mapping tells us precisely how love is being conceptualized as a journey. And this unified way of conceptualizing love metaphorically is realized in many different linguistic expressions.

In addition, we saw above that inference patterns from the

travel domain can be used to reason about love. Hence, metaphorical reasoning does exist. As to similarity, there is nothing inherently similar between love and journeys, yet they are linked metaphorically. Finally, all of the metaphorical expressions we looked at in the LOVE IS A JOURNEY metaphor are ordinary, everyday expressions rather than poetic or especially rhetorical expressions.

It should be noted that contemporary theorists commonly use the term *metaphor* to refer to the conceptual mapping, and the term *metaphorical expression* to refer to an individual linguistic expression (e.g., **dead-end street)** that is sanctioned by a mapping. We have adopted this terminology for the following reason: Metaphor, as a phenomenon, involves both conceptual mappings and individual linguistic expressions. It is important to keep them distinct. Since it is the mappings that are primary and that state the generalizations that are our principal concern, we have reserved the term *metaphor* for the mappings rather than for the linguistic expressions.

In the literature of the field, small capitals like LOVE IS A JOURNEY are used as mnemonics to name mappings. Thus, when we refer to the LOVE IS A JOURNEY metaphor, we are referring to the set of correspondences discussed above. The English sentence "Love is a journey," on the other hand, is a metaphorical expression that is understood via that set of correspondences.

# Generalizations

The LOVE IS A JOURNEY metaphor is a conceptual mapping that characterizes a generalization of two kinds:

- *Polysemy generalization:* A generalization over related senses of linguistic expressions—for example, **dead-end street, crossroads, stuck, spinning one's wheels, not going anywhere,** and so on.
- *Inferential generalization:* A generalization over inferences across different conceptual domains.

That is, the existence of the mapping provides a general answer to two questions:

- Why are words for travel used to describe love relationships?
- Why are inference patterns used to reason about travel also used to reason about love relationships?

Correspondingly, from the perspective of the linguistic analyst, the existence of such cross-domain pairings of words and of inference patterns provides evidence for the existence of such mappings.

## Novel Extensions of Conventional Metaphors

The fact that the LOVE IS A JOURNEY mapping is a fixed part of our conceptual system explains why new and imaginative uses of the mapping can be understood instantly, given the ontological correspondences and other knowledge about journeys. Take the song lyric,

> We're driving in the fast lane on the freeway of love.

The traveling knowledge called upon is this: When you drive in the fast lane, you go a long way in a short time and it can be exciting and dangerous. The general metaphorical mapping maps this knowledge about driving onto knowledge about love relationships. The danger may be to the vehicle (the relationship may not last) or to the passengers (the lovers may be hurt emotionally). The excitement of the love-journey is sexual. Our understanding of the song lyric is a consequence of the preexisting metaphorical correspondences of the LOVE IS A JOURNEY metaphor. The song lyric is instantly comprehensible to speakers of English because those metaphorical correspondences are already part of our conceptual system.

## Motivation

Each conventional metaphor, that is, each mapping, is a fixed pattern of conceptual correspondences across conceptual domains. As such, each mapping defines an open-ended class of potential correspondences across inference patterns. When activated, a mapping may apply to a novel source-domain knowledge structure and characterize a corresponding target-domain knowledge structure.

Mappings should not be thought of as processes, or as algorithms that mechanically take source-domain inputs and produce target-domain outputs. Instead, each mapping should be seen as a fixed pattern of ontological correspondences across domains that may or may not be applied to a source-domain knowledge structure or a source-domain lexical item. Thus, lexical items that are conventional in the source domain are not always conventional in the target domain. Instead, each source-domain lexical item may or may not make use of the static mapping pattern. If it does, it has an extended lexicalized sense in the target domain, where that sense is characterized by the mapping. If not, the source-domain lexical item will not have a conventional sense in the target domain, but may still be actively mapped in the case of novel metaphor. Thus, although the words *freeway* and *fast lane* are not conventionally used of love, the knowledge structures associated with these words are mapped by the LOVE IS A JOURNEY metaphor in the case of "We're driving in the fast lane on the freeway of love."

## Imagable Idioms

Many of the metaphorical expressions discussed in the literature on conventional metaphor are idioms. In the classical view, idioms have arbitrary meanings. But within cognitive linguistics, the possibility exists that idioms are motivated rather than arbitrary; that is, they do not arise automatically by productive rules, but they fit one or more patterns present in the conceptual system. Let us look a little more closely at idioms.

An idiom like "spinning one's wheels" comes with a conventional mental image, that of the wheels of a car stuck in some substance—in mud, sand, or snow, or on ice—so that the car cannot move when the motor is engaged and the wheels turn. Our knowledge about that image includes the following points: 1) a lot of energy is being used up (in spinning the wheels) without any progress being made; 2) the situation will not readily change of its own accord; and 3) it will take a lot of effort on the part of the occupants to get the vehicle moving again—and that may not even be possible.

The LOVE IS A JOURNEY metaphor applies to this knowledge about the image. It maps this knowledge onto knowledge about love relationships: A lot of energy is being spent without any progress toward fulfilling common goals, the situation will not change of its own accord, it will take a lot of effort on the part of the lovers to get the relationship moving again, and so on. In short, when idioms have associated conventional images, it is common for an independently motivated conceptual metaphor to map knowledge of those images from the source to the target domain. For a survey of experiments verifying the existence of such images and such mappings, see Gibbs 1994.

## Mappings at the Superordinate Level

In the LOVE IS A JOURNEY mapping, a love relationship corresponds to a vehicle. A vehicle is a superordinate category that includes such basic-level subcategories as car, train, boat, and plane. Indeed, the examples of vehicles are typically drawn from this range of basic-level categories: car (long, bumpy road; spinning our wheels), train (off the track), boat (on the rocks, foundering), plane (just taking off, bailing out). This is not an accident; in general, we have found that mappings are at the superordinate rather than the basic level. Thus, we would be surprised to find fully general submappings like A LOVE RELATIONSHIP IS A CAR; when we find a love relationship conceptualized as a car, we also tend to find it conceptualized as a boat, a train, a plane, and the like. It is the superordinate category VEHICLE, not the basic-level category CAR, that is in the general mapping in this case, and that is common in the system (although there may be instances in which this is not so).

It should be no surprise that the generalization is at the super-ordinate level whereas the special cases are at the basic level. After all, the basic level is the level of rich mental images and rich knowledge structure. (For a discussion of the properties of basic-level categories, see Lakoff 1987, pp. 31–50.) A mapping at the superordinate level maximizes the possibilities for mapping rich conceptual structure in the source domain onto the target domain, since it permits many basic-level instances, each of which is infor-mation rich.

Thus, a prediction is made about conventional mappings: the categories mapped will tend to be at the superordinate rather than the basic level. Thus, one tends not to find mappings like A LOVE RELATIONSHIP IS A CAR or A LOVE RELATIONSHIP IS A BOAT. Instead, one tends to find both basic-level cases (e.g., both cars and boats), which indicates that the generalization is one level higher, at the superordinate level of the vehicle. In most of the hundreds of cases of conventional mappings studied so far, it has been borne out that superordinate categories are used in mappings.

There are, however, occasional cases in which basic-level cate-gories seem to show up in mappings or uncertainty exists as to whether a particular category should be considered basic level. For example, anger is a basic emotion. Should it be considered a basic-level concept? There is no shortage of conceptual metaphors for anger: ANGER IS A HOT FLUID IN A CONTAINER, ANGER IS MAD-NESS, and so on. It is not clear whether anger should not be considered a basic-level category or a case in which a basic-level category occurs in a mapping. Another case will be discussed later in this chapter: The IMPOTENCE IS BLINDNESS metaphor (observed by Freud) contains a submapping, TESTICLES ARE EYES. This sub-mapping certainly involves basic-level concepts. It is not clear what significance, if any, this fact has for the theory of metaphor. There is nothing in the general theory that requires mappings to be on the superordinate level; it is simply an empirical fact that they tend to occur that way. This tendency may just follow from the fact that mappings at the superordinate level do more conceptual work than mappings at lower levels. It could be that mappings tend to be optimized for information content, but that occasional mappings at the basic level occur for other reasons—for example, when there is an experiential basis for a mapping at the basic level but not at the superordinate level.

In the remainder of this chapter, when I speak of a *metaphor* or a *conceptual metaphor*, I shall be referring to a mapping of the sort we have just discussed. With this example of a conceptual metaphor in place, let us turn to the relationship between conceptual metaphor and dreams.

## Metaphor and Dreams

What I have to say about dreams is not entirely new. The basic point goes back to a remark of Freud's in "The Interpretation of Dreams," in a discussion of dream symbolism (Freud 1900/1953, p. 351):

> [T]his symbolism is not peculiar to dreams, but is characteristic of unconscious ideation . . . and it is to be found in folklore, and in popular myths, legends, linguistic idioms, proverbial wisdom and current jokes, to a more complete extent than in dreams.

It is my job, as a linguist and a cognitive scientist, to study systematically what Freud called "unconscious ideation" of a symbolic nature. I specialize in the study of conceptual systems—the largely unconscious systems of thought in terms of which we think, and on which ordinary, everyday language is based. I do this largely on the basis of the systematic study of what Freud called "linguistic idioms."

What I and my colleagues have found, in a decade and a half of study, is that, as Freud suggested, we have systems of "unconscious ideation" of a symbolic nature. One of these is a very large system of conceptual metaphor and metonymy, and I and my colleagues and students have been tracing out this system in extensive detail. Freud was right when he suggested that this system is even more elaborately used in ordinary "linguistic idioms" than in dreams.

Having worked out a very large part of this system for English, I would like to show in some detail how it functions in dreams. Interestingly enough, Freud and other dream analysts have not already done this. Neither Freud nor other psychoanalysts have been interested in working out the details of the system of mundane, metaphorical thought, although they implicitly recognized the existence of such a mode of thought and have made implicit use of it as part of dream interpretation. The job of working out the details of the metaphor system has fallen to linguists and cognitive scientists. Freud and many of his followers were interested more in sexual symbolism—metaphors of a tabooed nature. But what we find through the study of everyday language is that unconscious symbolic thought is, for the most part, not sexual or tabooed. Tabooed thought only rarely shows up in ordinary, everyday, conventional language. What I will be doing is thus something that other dream analysts have not already done. It is, if anything, the tame part of dream analysis—the study of how unconscious symbolic thought of the most ordinary, nontabooed kind shows up in dreams.

The purpose of this chapter is to provide a set of examples of commonplace dreams in which our ordinary system of metaphor mediates between the overt content of the dream and the way we understand dreams as applying to our everyday lives. In the examples of dream interpretations that I will be discussing, conceptual metaphor plays the following role:

> Let **D** = the overt content of the dream. Let **M** = a collection of conceptual metaphors from our conceptual system. Let **K** = knowledge about the dreamer's history and everyday life. Let **I** = an interpretation of the dream in terms of the dreamer's life.

That is, **I** is the interpreted meaning of the dream, which the interpreter hopes he or she has accurately portrayed. The relationship between the dream and its interpretation is as follows:

$D \rightarrow I$, given $K$: Metaphors map the dream onto the interpretation of the dream, given relevant knowledge of the dreamer's life.

$D$ is what Freud called the "manifest content" of the dream, and $I$ is what he called the "latent content."

If this is correct, then the system of conceptual metaphor plays a critical role in the interpretation of dreams. However, it cannot be used in isolation, without knowledge of the dreamer's everyday life to yield a meaningful interpretation. This will become clear in the cases to be discussed below.

$I$, the interpretation of the dream, can be understood in two ways:

1. *The Weak Interpretation:* $I$ is the interpretation ascribed to the dream by an interpreter—either another party or the dreamer on conscious reflection.
2. *The Strong Interpretation:* $I$ is the hidden meaning of the dream to the dreamer.

The weak claim of this chapter is that our everyday system of conventional metaphor is employed whenever an interpreter interprets a dream. It is part of what defines a plausible interpretation. I believe I can demonstrate this beyond doubt.

But the stronger claim is more interesting: The metaphor system plays a generative role in dreaming—mediating between the meaning of the dream to the dreamer and what is seen, heard, and otherwise experienced dynamically in the act of dreaming. Given a meaning to be expressed, the metaphor system provides a means of expressing it concretely—in ways that can be seen and heard. That is, the metaphor system, which is in place for waking thought and expression, is also available during sleep and provides a natural mechanism for relating concrete images to abstract meanings. Of course, upon waking, the dreamer may well not be aware of the meaning of the dream, since he or she did not consciously direct the choice of dream imagery to metaphorically express the meaning of the dream.

The stronger claim is harder to demonstrate, and I cannot demonstrate it by the methods of the linguist. At best I can make a plausible case for it by providing plausible interpretations—interpretations of what the dream can plausibly have meant to the dreamer, given the concerns of his or her everyday life.

Before we proceed, several points need to be made.

**First,** it is important to clarify what I mean by *unconscious* in the expression "unconscious conceptual system." Freud used the term to mean thoughts that were repressed but might in some cases be brought to consciousness. But the term *unconscious* is used very differently in the cognitive sciences. Most of the kinds of thought discussed in the cognitive sciences operate, like the rules of grammar and phonology, below a level that we could possibly have conscious access to or control over.

It is possible, through linguistic analysis, to discover what metaphors one uses in unconscious thought, and to discuss these overtly. For example, one might discover that one thinks in terms of the LOVE IS A JOURNEY metaphor, and then have a discussion about the way one has used the metaphor. But there is no way to achieve conscious control over all unconscious uses of that metaphor and other metaphors in one's conceptual system. It is like consciously discussing a rule of grammar or phonology without being able to control all the rules of one's grammar and phonology in every sentence one speaks. The system of metaphors, although unconscious, is not "repressed"—just as the system of grammatical and phonological rules that structure one's language is unconscious but not repressed. The unconscious discovered by cognitive science is just not like the Freudian unconscious.

**Second,** the interpretations I will be offering may well seem obvious or pedestrian. Indeed, that is their point. The everyday metaphor system characterizes the most normal and natural of interpretations. My purpose is to say exactly why there are normal, natural interpretations of dreams. As a consequence, I will be starting where most dream analysts end. Most dream analysts are satisfied when they arrive at an intuitively plausible interpretation of a dream. I will be starting with intuitively plausible analyses and trying to show exactly what makes them intuitively plausible.

**Third,** as I said above, I cannot prove that the analyses I will be giving are the "right" ones, nor that they are the only ones. What I claim to show is that they are yielded by the metaphor system given a choice of **K**, a selected portion of knowledge of the dreamer's everyday life. A different choice of relevant knowledge, **K'**, could produce a completely different interpretation.

**Fourth,** I assume that dreaming is a form of thought. Powerful dreams are forms of thought that express emotionally powerful content. Two of the main discoveries of cognitive science are that most thought is unconscious and that most thought makes use of conceptual metaphor. Dreams are also a form of unconscious thought that makes use of conceptual metaphor. As a form of thought, dreams can express content: desires, fears, solutions to problems, fantasies, and so on. If Freud was right in suggesting that something like repression exists, that there are some thoughts that we don't want to be aware that we are thinking, then the use of the conscious metaphor system in dreams is a perfect way for the unconscious mind to hide thoughts from the conscious mind while nonetheless thinking them.

**Fifth,** dreams are a form of thought, and they make use of metaphor because thought typically makes use of metaphor. Since dreams are not consciously monitored, they do not make consciously monitored use of metaphor. Thus, the use of metaphor in dreams may seem to the conscious mind wild and incoherent.

**Sixth,** the imagery used in dreams is not arbitrary; rather, it is constrained by the general metaphors used by the dreamer. The general metaphors are sets of correlations between source and target domains at the superordinate level. Dream imagery is chosen from the basic (and subordinate) level—that is, from special cases of superordinate categories characterized by the general metaphors.

For example, suppose a dream is about love. One of the metaphors for love will be used in the dream. If it is LOVE IS A JOURNEY, then the dream imagery will be about a particular kind of journey, say, a car trip. Then the dream images might include a car, roads, bridges, bad weather, and so forth. Because metaphorical thought is natural, the use of images in dream thought is also natural.

**Seventh,** I therefore claim that dreams are not just the weird and meaningless product of random neural firings, but rather a natural way by which emotionally charged fears, desires, and descriptions of difficulties in life are expressed.

Incidentally, what I am claiming is consistent with the claim that dreams are set off by random neural firings in the brain stem. It is possible that a fixed, conventional metaphor system could channel random neural firings into a meaningful dream. In other words, if dreams turn out to be triggered by random neural firings, it would not necessarily follow that the content of dreams is random.

**Eighth,** dreaming is a process with open-ended possibilities for metaphorical expression. What those possibilities are is determined by the fixed, general metaphors in the conceptual system. The fixed metaphors are fixed correspondences across conceptual domains at the superordinate level. Those fixed correspondences make it possible for basic-level imagery to have systematic meaning. Since the possibilities for basic- and subordinate-level imagery are open ended, the fixed metaphorical correspondences allow for an open-ended range of possibilities in a particular dream. Dream construction is a dynamic process that makes use of fixed metaphorical correspondences to construct the image sequences that occur in dreams.

Thus, there is a sense in which dreaming is like speaking. We have fixed rules of grammar and phonology that constrain what sentences we can construct and what they can mean. But the rules, being general, permit an open-ended range of special cases that fit the rules. Similarly, our metaphor system might be seen as part of a "grammar of the unconscious"—a set of fixed, general principles that permit an open-ended range of possible dreams that are constructed dynamically in accordance with those principles. To understand the system of metaphor is to understand those principles.

**Ninth,** I claim that deep and extensive knowledge of the dreamer's life is essential to pinpointing the meanings of dreams. Does that mean that dreams cannot have interpretations on their own, independent of what we know about the dreamer?

Well, yes and no. There is a certain well-demarcated range of typical emotional concerns in this culture: love, work, death, family, and the like. It is a good bet that powerful dreams will be about one of those domains. This puts a constraint on what the target domains of metaphors are likely to be. Suppose each interpretation of a dream concerns one of those domains. That means one can fix a single domain to be the target domain for all of the metaphorical images used in the dream. The metaphor system allows each metaphorical image to have a wide range of interpretations. But if the dream is a long sequence of metaphorical images, then the choice of a single target domain limits the possibilities for interpretation of the whole collection of images. Thus, it might be possible to narrow the range of possible interpretations for a given dream without knowledge of the dreamer.

But even such a narrowed range of possibilities might be extremely large—so large that one could not even come close to imagining the range of possibilities. Two mechanisms make even such a narrowed range of possibilities very large. First, the range of specific instances of a general metaphor could be extremely broad. Second, what Turner and I (Lakoff and Turner 1989) have called the GENERIC IS SPECIFIC metaphor schema allows for an open-ended range of metaphorical correspondences across domains. The use of this metaphor schema (described below) depends on detailed knowledge. These two mechanisms allow for such a broad range of possibilities that only detailed knowledge of the life of the dreamer can limit that range of possibilities to what the dream means to that dreamer.

It should be said, however, that the wide range of possibilities permits an individual dream to have multiple meanings for a dreamer, and I claim that especially powerful dreams commonly have multiple meanings.

In addition, because of the wide range of possibilities permitted by the metaphor system, one person's dreams can have powerful meanings for other people. Other people's dreams hold for us the same fascination as myth and literature—a potential vehicle for finding meaning in our own lives. It is the operation of our metaphor systems that allows such a possibility.

The dream analyses to follow stress the importance of deep and extensive knowledge about the life of the dreamer. In each case, I have used a dream of someone I know very well, and it is only because I know the dreamer well that I feel confident of the interpretations.

## The Anthropologist's Dream

A woman I will call Maggie dreamed that she starting hiking on a pleasant, wide, well-paved road. After a while, the road narrowed, turned to a dirt road, and started winding through the brush. The road got narrower and narrower and the terrain became rough, and soon she found herself climbing uphill, sliding, passing through heavy brush, pushing branches aside, and barely able to move along the trail at all. Exhausted, she reached a clearing at the top of the hill. There she saw a friend of hers coming out of Trader Joe's, the market where local academics buy their gourmet foods. "Don't bother," he said, "The anthropologists have cleared it all out."

Maggie is an anthropologist. After many years of graduate school, fieldwork, and raising a family, she finally wrote her thesis and got her Ph.D. At the time she had started graduate school, there were abundant academic jobs for anthropologists. But by the time she finally got her degree, most of the jobs were taken. For years she took part-time jobs at various places, hoping to get a full-time job, but with no success.

At the time of the dream, she had finally given up on anthropology and was starting out on a new career. Trader Joe's, in the city where she lives, is where the local academics go to buy the amenities of life: imported cheeses, wines, and so on.

The conventional metaphor that structures this dream is called the EVENT STRUCTURE metaphor. It has a number of parts, among them the following:

- STATES ARE LOCATIONS
- ACTIONS ARE SELF-PROPELLED MOTIONS
- PURPOSES ARE DESTINATIONS

- MEANS ARE PATHS
- DIFFICULTIES ARE IMPEDIMENTS TO MOTION

The STATES ARE LOCATIONS metaphor is used in expressions such as "She is in love" or "He is out of his depression." PURPOSES ARE DESTINATIONS lies behind the use of the word "goal" to express a purpose. It occurs in expressions such as **"reaching one's goals,"** **"falling short** of one's expectations," **"progressing,"** and so on. The use of the PATH word *way* (as in "Go about it any **way** you want") to express the means of achieving a purpose is an instance of MEANS ARE PATHS. Thus, action designed to achieve a purpose is conceptualized in this metaphor as self-propelled motion along a path toward a destination. Difficulties in achieving one's purpose are naturally conceptualized as impediments to motion: things that make it harder to move—namely, things that get in one's way, features of the terrain, burdens that weigh one down, and so on.

A second metaphor for achieving a purpose enters into the dream, namely,

- ACHIEVING A PURPOSE IS EATING

Thus, we can **"smell** success," "be so close we can **taste** it," and enjoy the **"fruits** of our labor."

Much of the dream is an instance of DIFFICULTIES ARE IMPEDIMENTS TO MOTION. In the dream, Maggie's PURPOSE/DESTINATION is to get a university job as an anthropologist. The path to such a job, which started out wide and easy to walk on, is long, gets narrower and more winding, becomes covered with brush, and goes uphill. Maggie encounters difficulties, conceptualized as impediments to motion. She finally reaches the top of the hill—the top of the academic ladder, the Ph.D.—where she expects to be able to have desired objects—academic jobs—available to her. These are symbolized in the dreams by a metonymy in which food representing academic success—imported cheeses and wines— stands for the academic jobs. In her town, that food is at Trader Joe's. "The anthropologists have cleaned it out" indicates that no food/jobs are left.

## The Blindness Dream

A man I will call Steve had the recurring dream that he had become blind. He would awaken his wife in the middle of night, hysterically screaming, "I'm blind, I'm blind," until his wife could wake him up, turn on the light, and show him that he could see.

Steve is a scrupulous, meticulous, and cautious academic who is always afraid that he doesn't know enough. In our everyday conceptual system, there is a metaphor—KNOWING IS SEEING—that appears in everyday expressions such as

> I **see** what you're getting at. His meaning was **clear.** You can't **pull the wool over my eyes.** This paragraph is a bit **murky.** What is your **viewpoint?**

Via this metaphor, "I can't see" maps onto "I don't know—and can't find out." Steve, in his dream, is expressing his constant fear: "I'm ignorant, I'm ignorant."

But Steve's dream, as a powerful, recurrent dream, is richer than that. Freud, in his interpretation of the Oedipus myth, observed that Oedipus' gouging out of his eyes was a metaphorical castration, the metaphor being that TESTICLES ARE EYES and IMPOTENCE IS BLINDNESS. By virtue of this metaphor, being blinded is a just punishment for a sexual transgression. It is because this metaphor is in our conceptual system that we understand Oedipus' punishment as being just. Incidentally, contemporary popular culture also has a manifestation of this metaphor in the folk theory that if you masturbate, you'll go blind.

A linguistic expression of this metaphor appeared in the *San Francisco Chronicle* during the trial of Elly Nessler in the California Gold Country north of Sacramento. During the trial of a man who was accused of molesting her young son, Nessler came into the courtroom with a gun and shot the defendant in the head, killing him. Nessler subsequently stood trial for the man's murder. While covering the proceedings, a *Chronicle* reporter asked a local citizen what he thought of Nessler's deed. The man replied, "I'd have aimed lower and shot his eyes out." To the millions of readers of the *Chronicle* in the Bay Area, the TESTICLES ARE EYES metaphor was immediately understandable.

One of the banes of Steve's existence is the feeling that he lacks power and influence, and is therefore unable to fulfill the needs of himself and others. Steve's blindness dream recurred several times just before he took on his first important administrative position, a job in which he feared he would expend a great deal of energy yet fail to accomplish anything of significance. We have a common cultural metaphor that WORLDLY POWER IS SEXUAL PO-TENCY and POWERLESSNESS IS IMPOTENCE.

Linguistic examples of this metaphor abound in everyday life. One of the most celebrated was Lyndon Johnson's remark about a political enemy whom he had the power to blackmail: "I've got his pecker in my pocket." Men threatening to get back at an enemy by rendering him powerless have been heard to say "I'll cut his balls off" or "I'll castrate him." Women who exert worldly power over men are regularly called "castrating bitches."

Via this metaphor, "I'm blind" in the dream expresses another of Steve's recurrent fears: "I'm powerless."

In addition, the dream has still further significance for Steve's life. Steve cannot have children because of a low sperm count. After years of trying to have children, Steve and his wife finally adopted and are now happy and loving parents. Still, it was a traumatic experience in Steve's life to learn that he would not be able to have biological children. Via the metaphor of IMPOTENCE IS BLINDNESS, when Steve cries out, "I'm blind," he is expressing that trauma. Metaphorically, he is crying out, "I'm impotent."

Steve's recurrent dream is powerful because it expresses three of the major fears and regrets of his life. Metaphor is the mecha-nism that links the dream to its meaning. What makes this dream extremely powerful is that it has not one but three simultaneous metaphorical meanings via three different metaphors. Two of these metaphors are expressed in everyday language: Both KNOW-ING IS SEEING and WORLDLY POWER IS SEXUAL POTENCY are part of the largely unconscious system of metaphorical thought that un-derlies much of our everyday language. GENITALS ARE EYES and IMPOTENCE IS BLINDNESS, on the other hand, have a very different status, in that they represent an unconscious conceptual metaphor that, although widespread in our culture, is tabooed. Thus, aside from the isolated case cited above, there is no large set of everyday linguistic expressions that are comprehended via this metaphor. For example, "My eyes hurt" does not mean "My testicles hurt," and "He's blind" does not mean " He's impotent."

Yet the metaphor seems to be present nonetheless, and there is a good reason why it should be—it has the right kind of experiential basis to form a metaphor—namely, testicles are the same shape as eyes, and losing one's eyesight renders one relatively powerless. The existence of such an experiential basis for the metaphor makes the metaphor natural. Apparently, the IMPO-TENCE IS BLINDNESS metaphor, though tabooed and unrealized in everyday language, is part of our conceptual systems. If it weren't, the Oedipus myth would seem senseless since blindness, in the absence of such a metaphor, would not seem a just punishment for incest. Several theoretical morals arise from this set of interpretations of the Blindness Dream:

**First,** Freudian symbolism (as when the eyes symbolize genitals) can have the status of a tabooed metaphor that, despite having no reflection in everyday linguistic expressions, is just as psychically real as other conceptual metaphors.

**Second,** tabooed metaphors (with no reflection in language) such as EYES ARE GENITALS and IMPOTENCE IS BLINDNESS may combine with nontabooed metaphors such as WORLDLY POWER IS SEX-UAL POTENCY to jointly provide an interpretation of a dream. In short, much of Freud's symbolism is in the form of tabooed metaphors that—rather than being segregated from—can be combined with everyday, nontabooed metaphors.

**Third,** a dream can have multiple, simultaneous interpretations, all of which are equally valid. It is natural for a powerful, recurrent dream to have such multiple meanings.

## The Bridge Dream

A man I will call Herb fell in love and moved in with his girlfriend. Moving in turned out to be a disaster. They simply could not live together without fighting. With great sadness, they decided to split up. The night they came to this decision, Herb dreamed that as they started out on a trip from Berkeley, a fierce storm blew up, and as they reached the Richmond–San Raphael Bridge (across the San Francisco Bay), the bridge blew away into the bay.

This dream uses two common conventional metaphors. The first is the EMOTIONAL CLIMATE metaphor, in which INTERIOR EMOTIONS ARE EXTERIOR WEATHER CONDITIONS. Thus, a happy person has a sunny disposition, and happiness is light, whereas sadness and depression are dark. A special case of this metaphor is EMOTIONAL DISCORD IS A STORM. Via this metaphor, the storm symbolized the emotional discord of the fighting involved in the lovers' breakup.

The other metaphor involved is LOVE IS A JOURNEY. Setting out on the journey corresponds to the long-term commitment made by the lovers when they moved in together. The washing out of the bridge, which made it impossible to continue the journey, corresponds to the ending of the love relationship. Without the bridge, the journey could not continue. The washing out of the bridge has a second meaning via another common metaphor, in which RELATIONSHIPS ARE LINKS BETWEEN PEOPLE. Here the falling away of the bridge indicates the end of the relationship link between the lovers.

## The Flying Dreams

A man I will call David always does things to extremes, whether working or having fun. He tries to live as joyous and fulfilling a life as possible. He works as a lawyer, primarily on cases that he believes in, and spends very long hours, often for months at a time, wearing himself out. He is also a musician who likes to play far into the night or go to late-night concerts and party for long hours. He loves the outdoors and will drive for many hours each way to go skiing for the weekend. He takes long, vigorous walks and bike rides. He is generally happy, but when he exhausts himself, he becomes gaunt and sick and depressed.

David has long had recurring dreams in which he was flying. In his early 20s, he would fly too high or fast or far in his dreams and become terrified. Then he took a chance and did something he had always wanted to do. He went to Paris, worked as a street singer, made a lot of friends, and had a wonderful time. At this point, he had a flying dream in which he flew especially high and fast, got scared, feared crashing, landed on the shoulders of a friend, did a backflip into the air, and landed on his feet. Thereafter, his dreams of flying were pleasurable. He has been confident ever since that he would land on his feet.

The common metaphors involved are these:

- ACTION IS SELF-PROPELLED MOTION
- FREEDOM IS LACK OF CONSTRAINT
- INTENSE ACTION IS FAST MOTION

Flying, in this metaphor, is a form of fast motion with no constraints, but with the danger of falling and crashing, which signifies resulting harm. Metaphorically, flying is intense action with a sense of freedom—what David prizes most. The flying dreams accompanied periods of intense action in the service of freedom—driving a taxicab in Boston after college, street-singing in Paris, working as a lawyer for idealistic causes, putting together a band and making tapes and a video, and going off on vigorous and exciting vacation trips.

In Paris, where he found the help of friends, the flying dream was extended by the metaphor of HELP IS SUPPORT—he landed on a friend's shoulders. Then he did a backflip (a form of playful showing off) and landed on his feet (signifying a safe result). Indeed, we have the idiom "to land on one's feet" in English, which works by the same metaphors.

## The Time Bomb Dream

A woman I will call Eileen dreamed that she was observing a mule having brain surgery. The mule's head was cut open and a time bomb was placed inside. The mule was then stitched up and ran off, becoming a beautiful, graceful horse. Eileen watches in terror as the horse prances gracefully with a time bomb in its head.

To comprehend this dream, the following information is necessary:

- Our cultural stereotype of the mule is that it is 1) stubborn, 2) sterile, and 3) clumsy compared with the horse.
- Eileen is in love with a man whom she wants to marry. She has a grown child by a former marriage, and at her age, with her biological clock ticking, she is not likely to have any children in her second marriage. This upsets her.
- She is also very determined about how she wants to live her life. She wants to pursue a particular career, and at this point in her life, she feels the clock is running out on her. She will have to start soon.
- Moreover, the way she had always assumed she would pursue a career conflicts with her plans for marriage. Indeed, a number of her plans and desires conflict with the marriage that she very much wants. Thus, she is pursuing inconsistent desires.
- Eileen is a worrier and has a history of panic attacks. For some years, she was on medication to prevent such attacks, but had been off the medicine for several months at the time of the dream. Just before the dream, she had a panic attack and wound up in an argument with her prospective husband about her conflicting desires. She fears further panic attacks.
- Eileen went into therapy 4 years before the dream, at a time when she was barely functioning because of the panic attacks. When she entered therapy, she had just broken off a damaging long-term relationship and had difficulty dealing with men as well as functioning professionally. Through therapy, she reached a point where she could function well again. She established a good relationship with the man she wants to marry and was able to return to her professional goals.
- Eileen is also a former dancer who takes joy in physical activity, especially in her regular aerobics class. She counts on physical activity to keep her healthy and stable. And her

excellent physical shape makes her constantly aware that she is still capable of having children.

The mechanisms relating Eileen's dream to her life are the GREAT CHAIN OF BEING metaphor schema (Lakoff and Turner 1989) and one of the major metaphors for ideas—IDEAS ARE OBJECTS IN THE MIND.

According to the IDEAS ARE OBJECTS metaphor, ideas move in the direction of their consequences. Thus, following an idea entails being led to its consequences. Ideas with inconsistent consequences are thus moving in opposite directions. They exert force on each other, and are thus seen as being in conflict.

The GREAT CHAIN metaphor schema makes use of a folk version of the "Great Chain of Being," in which there is a hierarchy of beings, with humans at the top, higher animals below them, and lower animals, plants, and inanimate objects further down. The metaphor schema is a mechanism by which human behavior is understood in terms of the behavior of forms of being lower on the chain. The metaphor works by metaphorically attributing to humans the distinguishing properties of beings lower on the chain. The being lower on the Great Chain is the mule; its distinguishing properties are stubbornness, sterility, and clumsiness (relative to horses).

Eileen was metaphorically a mule before therapy (an operation on her head), which enabled her to function well, to transform from a mule to a gracefully prancing horse. But she retains the inherent properties of a mule: stubbornness and sterility. She is stubborn about how she wants to live her life; sterile, in that she will not be having any children in her future marriage. The conflicting desires—her desire for marriage and her career aspirations—were restored to her through therapy, the operation on her head. But the desires conflict—they exert force on one another inside her head and have a potential to metaphorically explode. They constitute the time bomb in her head. The time bomb also symbolizes her biological clock and her career clock, and the possibility of explosion symbolizes the destruction of her hopes of having more children and of pursuing a career. The possible return of panic attacks symbolizes another kind of metaphorical explosion. Meanwhile, in joyful physical activity, functioning in a good relationship, and pursuing her career, she is the graceful horse—with a time bomb in her head!

# Conclusion

It should be clear by now that our everyday metaphor system shapes our dreams, allowing for the expression—in another (perhaps "safer") form—of our deepest difficulties and anxieties.

Conventional metaphors have the potential to link concrete imagery, especially visual imagery, to more abstract concepts. Since the metaphor system is a fixed part of our unconscious system of concepts, conventional metaphors are always available to link concrete imagery to abstract meanings. And given abstract meanings, the metaphor system can constrain the choice of concrete imagery appropriate to express those meanings. As a result, the concerns of everyday life can be expressed via concrete imagery plus metaphors. Our system of conceptual metaphor makes it possible to express desires, fears, and characterizations of emotionally charged situations.

The metaphor system of English is now being studied systematically and scientifically. The result is a kind of dictionary of unconscious thought. In general, the metaphor system shared by members of a culture can be thought of as having two parts: 1) the ordinary, conventional metaphors, which, although unconscious, have reflexes in everyday language; and 2) the tabooed metaphors, which, because of their tabooed nature, are not expressed in conventional language. Freud, because of his concern with sexuality and repression, was largely concerned with tabooed metaphors. I, because I am a linguist by profession, am largely concerned with the everyday metaphors that show up in ordinary language.

Because dream interpretation has largely been done by psychotherapists, the kinds of analyses I have discussed, although certainly noticed, have never been the subject of systematic and rigorous study. But now that linguistics and cognitive science have yielded an understanding of our everyday metaphor system, it has become possible to apply that knowledge to dream interpretation in a systematic way.

The everyday, nontabooed metaphors are every bit as important to the understanding of dreams as the tabooed ones. Some therapists have an instinctive understanding of how our everyday metaphor system operates in dreams. But many do not. When I read books on dream analysis by psychotherapists, I rarely find much attention accorded to those aspects of the meanings of dreams that depend on the everyday metaphor system.

The metaphor system is far from obvious. Those who want to make use of it in dream interpretation should probably obtain some training in how the system works. After all, if one is using the language of the unconscious, it might be useful to get a few grammar lessons and have a dictionary handy.

I would like to conclude by discussing what I am not claiming. I am not, for example, promoting a new form of dream therapy. I am certainly not claiming that metaphor analysis replaces other forms of dream work in therapy. The metaphor system will inevitably be used in any form of dream work, simply because we use that system whenever we think. But the metaphor system does not determine what form the dream work should take. For example, Fritz Perls introduced into gestalt therapy the technique of having the dreamer take on the role of every person and thing in the dream. In doing so, dreamers will almost without exception make some or other use of their everyday metaphor systems; however, the power of the therapeutic technique is not in the use of the metaphor system per se. As with poetry in a foreign language, one needs to use a dictionary, but the poetry constitutes far more than what is in the dictionary.

Although this chapter has been about dreams, it should be clear that metaphor analysis can be useful in every aspect of psychotherapy. People can believe their metaphors and live according to them. Moreover, early childhood experience can serve as a metaphorical source for adult life, as Freud observed. Systematic training in metaphor analysis would, I believe, be enormously useful as part of the training of any psychotherapist.

# References

Damasio A: Descartes' Error: Emotion, Reason, and the Human Brain. New York, Putnam, 1994

Freud S: The interpretation of dreams (1900), in Standard Edition of the Complete Psychological Works of Sigmund Freud, Vols 4 and 5. Translated and edited by Strachey J. London, Hogarth Press, 1953

Gibbs RW Jr: The Poetics of Mind: Figurative Thought, Language and Understanding. Cambridge, UK, Cambridge University Press, 1994

Kövecses Z: Emotion Concepts. New York, Springer-Verlag, 1990

Lakoff G: Women, Fire, and Dangerous Things: What Categories Reveal About the Mind. Chicago, IL, University of Chicago Press, 1987

Lakoff G, Johnson M: Metaphors We Live By. Chicago, IL, University of Chicago Press, 1980

Lakoff G, Turner M: More Than Cool Reason. Chicago, IL, University of Chicago Press, 1989

# Chapter 5

# *What Neural Network Studies Suggest Regarding the Boundary Between Conscious and Unconscious Mental Processes*

Ralph Hoffman, M.D.

T he attention of neuroscientists has turned increasingly to the cooperative behavior of large ensembles of neurons (Gevins et al. 1987; Grey et al. 1989; Jenkins et al. 1990; Montgomery et al. 1992; Skarda and Freeman 1987). These empirical studies have been complemented by the development of computerized simulations of information processing by artificial neural networks. Capabilities for memory, perception, and cognition—albeit primitive— have been re-created with such models. The mind-brain problem remains daunting but has become, at least in principle, fathomable (Churchland and Sejnowski 1988).

In this chapter, I review the research in this area in terms of what it might say about unconscious mental processes. At first glance, my approach may seem backwards because I begin by discussing what studies of neural network processes suggest regarding the neurobiological basis of conscious mental processes. However, by exclusion, starting with this topic enables me to propose hypotheses regarding the neurobiology of mental processes that are not conscious.

For studies of neural networks to say anything useful at all about the biological mechanisms of conscious and unconscious mental processes is a very tall order. Discrete neural networks, both biological and simulated, are not obviously "conscious" in the ordinary sense of the word. In fact, asking whether ensembles of neurons are conscious might appear to reflect a kind of categorical error, like asking whether books are intelligent. On the other hand, it seems quite clear that our conscious experience—and the boundary between conscious and unconscious mental process-es—emerges from nothing more (or less) than a very complex neural network (i.e, the central nervous system).

# The Phenomenology of Conscious Experience

I begin by discussing phenomenological characteristics of con-scious experience in order to identify aspects of biological and simulated networks that demonstrate characteristics that parallel phenomenological characteristics of conscious experience. These parallels, in turn, may provide clues regarding aspects of neuronal network behavior that are correlates of conscious experience.

**First, consciousness always is consciousness of something.** Sensory impressions of the external world obviously form the basis of much conscious experience. What about conscious experi-ences that are generated internally? How do I know that I am thinking of a particular person? I "see" an image of that person in my mind, or say his or her name (Wittgenstein 1980a). Indeed, we can experience internally generated images involving one or more of all five sensory realms. We can "see" a tree in our minds and "hear" a voice or a piece of music as well as imagine the aroma of coffee, the feel of velvet on the forearm, or the sensation of hitting a strong tennis backhand. All are different kinds of inter-nally generated images that re-access representational capabilities emerging from the senses.

The other obvious constituent of conscious experience is emo-tion. Besides the basic emotions, perhaps analogous to the basic colors of the visual spectrum (happy, sad, angry, anxious), there are a range of complex emotions that constitute the full spectrum of coloration of our conscious lives (Gelernter 1994). Whimsy, loneliness, and wistfulness are examples.

One factor differentiating emotions from sensations is that the former, when considered alone, do not provide particular information about the external world but can provide a great deal of information about the internal state of one's mind. For example, the emotion anger does not say who I am angry at, whereas a mental image of a person immediately reflects the fact that I am thinking about that person—but may say little about how I am thinking about that person. Emotions such as anger or pleasure tell us that we are disposed to certain types of attitudes, expectations, and actions pertaining to the person.

The bottom line is that—leaving aside certain unusual states such as meditation—we are never conscious of nothing. Conscious experience always involves representations that reflect imagery and/or sensations that are either internally or externally generated, in combination with emotions—either simple (e.g., fear, happiness) or complex (e.g., wishes, urges, longings).

Many people would object to this rather limited view of consciousness. What about attitudes, beliefs, and intentions that can have no specific sensory or emotive content? For instance, what do I consciously experience when I am aware that I am a Democrat, an abstract concept devoid of a particular sensory referent which seems nonetheless apprehensible? How do I become conscious of this concept? My introspection reveals that I can feel a sense of kinship (a certain emotion) associated with a visual memory of Robert Kennedy. I remember whom I voted for in 1992. This remembrance has its own particulars: memories of seeing the names of candidates on the ballot, of pulling the voting lever, of telling friends, and so forth. I can remind myself of memories of certain political positions that I took during discussions with friends. I can anticipate how I might comment or argue in response to future political arguments. However, no matter how hard I try, I cannot access a direct experience of the abstract concept of being a Democrat. This abstraction, like others, needs to be instantiated by sensory and emotive particulars—or via actions in the present—in order to be experienced directly. This is not to say that these generalities and abstractions are not critical to our mental lives. They direct what elements are grouped together in our "stream of consciousness" as well as determine the objectives of our actions. The coherence of these thoughts and actions—bequeathed by common objectives—is perhaps what is recognizable as my "self": I recognize my actions and conscious thoughts as my own because they cohere with recognizable objectives.

Another tool that we use to become conscious of attitudes, beliefs, and other abstract concepts is language. We say words to ourselves or to others (or words are said to us) that express these concepts. However, this class of conscious experience, once again, is instantiated by external or imagistic activation of one of the senses—namely, by "hearing" the words that stand for these concepts. I can say to myself the word "Democrat," and experience it as a word. However, it has no particular experiential meaning except via the kinds of associations mentioned above or via its use in sentences that I say inwardly to myself or outwardly to others. But again, inescapably, saying words inwardly or outwardly produces a particular sensory experience—namely, the experience of a certain action (i.e., hearing oneself speak) or "hearing" an internal acoustic image of oneself speaking. Also, emotions are probably underestimated in terms of their importance in experiencing abstract concepts. For instance, the belief that the United States is a great country might be consciously experienced by, for instance, visually imagining our flag or a map of our country while simultaneously experiencing the emotion of pride. Other apparently abstract mentations, such as intending-to-act, can also be broken down into particular sensations, images, and emotions (Hoffman and Kravitz 1987). What constitutes consciousness of my intending to reach for a glass of water? Introspection suggests that I am actually referring to a complex interweaving of experiences that include the anticipatory proprioceptive image of the movement of the arm, the discomfort of thirst, the anticipatory image of drinking sensations, the emotion of desire, and so forth. The "glue" that holds all of these experiences together is their coherence and relevance to the intended act of drinking a glass of water. We are not directly conscious of the latter, however, in the abstract. We can say to ourselves, "I want to drink some water," but this, again, is an instantiation of inner speech, a kind of acoustic image. An alternative way to consciously experience wanting to drink water is by the act of reaching for the glass of water itself (a complex combination of proprioceptive and tactile sensations).

These simple introspections suggest that a necessary condition for a conscious experience—even when involving abstract concepts or intentions—is that one or more imagistic/perceptual or emotional systems encode meaningful information. It is widely held that emotions are experienced as bodily sensations (for an excellent review, see Papanicolaou 1989). Insofar as the other domain of consciousness consists of sensory representations—either externally driven or internally generated—the following hypothesis suggests itself:

> A necessary condition for conscious experience is meaningful encoding of information by brain areas responsible for somatic or sensory representations.

**Second, consciousness seems to occupy a continuous duration of time rather than consisting of a set of mental flash cards.** When we are visually conscious of a fork, sense data corresponding to "fork-ness" have been apprehended as a gestalt. As our eyes sweep over the fork, there is no disjunction of form; we experience a single fork, uninterrupted by blinks and saccades. Continuity over time seems to be a characteristic of all conscious object apprehension. Traditional studies of stimulus detection characterized critical stimulus duration thresholds for perception. Longer stimulus durations are generally required in order to perceive more complex stimuli (Dennett 1991). Sometimes the temporal organization of consciousness plays a trick on us. This trick of consciousness is exemplified by movie projection. A series of pictures are flashed at discrete intervals. However, our consciousness melds these flashes into a unity of objects and movements that appear seamless over time.

The most exemplary aspect of consciousness occurring over time is emotion. Emotional experience clearly has a duration, lasting from seconds to hours or longer. "Rage flares up, abates, vanishes; and likewise joy, depression, fear" (Wittgenstein 1980b, p. 28). Sorrow or anxiety can seem interminable. In light of the apparent temporal aspects of consciousness, I propose an addition to the hypothesis stated above:

> A necessary condition for conscious experience is meaningful encoding of information, by brain areas responsible for somatic or sensory representations, *that is sustained over a critical interval of time.*

This is not to say that other "association" brain areas not specifically dedicated to sensation or emotion cannot be active and sustained during conscious experience. I am proposing only that engagement of such brain areas alone is *not sufficient* for conscious experience to take place.

## A Thumbnail Sketch of Neural Network Information-Processing Models

Artificial neural network simulations are composed of large numbers of very simple computing units, generally referred to as "neurons," which are densely interconnected and transmit information according to "synaptic weights." These weights have numerical values that are either positive (i.e., excitatory) or negative (i.e., inhibitory) in nature. There is no single "command" unit or module; the effectiveness of the network as a whole reflects the cooperative interactions of its parts. Each neuron simultaneously receives information from a large number of other neurons and computes its response to these inputs in parallel with the computations of the other neurons of the system.

Of special relevance to this discussion are artificial networks that work on the basis of *attractor dynamics* (Amit 1989; Hinton and Shallice 1991; Hoffman 1987; Hopfield 1982; Smolensky 1986). The information-processing capabilities of these networks derive from the fact that they are "attracted to" particular activation patterns—namely, those representing the "low energy" states of the system. Here "energy" does not equate with the metabolic activation of the neural network but derives from a branch of physics known as statistical mechanics. Statistical mechanics has been used, for instance, to understand how magnetic moments of iron atoms interact to form a complex lattice. When magnetic moments of a group of proximal iron atoms align themselves in the same direction, the system is less disordered and has a lower statistical energy. When these magnetic moments are in disarray, statistical energy is increased. In general, statistical energy corresponds to the degree of disorder in the system.

For attractor-type neural networks, disorder at a particular time reflects the degree to which all pairs of neurons coactivate according to their connectivity weights. For instance, assume that neuron $i$ and neuron $j$ belong to a neural network. If these two neurons project to each other with excitatory connections, and both neurons are, at time $t$, either simultaneously active or simultaneously inactive, then the "energy" of the system will decrease. If this is not the case (i.e., if one neuron is activated while the other neuron is deactivated), then energy will increase. The overall energy of the system reflects the energy contribution of each pair of neurons and their connection weights. In general, the network as a whole always flows from higher to lower energy levels and seeks to stabilize at an energy minimum or attractor.

A new input into the system—which induces a new activation pattern among the neurons of the network—induces a new state of disorder. The system, in response, seeks another energy minimum or attractor that more or less incorporates the new pattern of activation induced by the new input. Neural networks tend, therefore, to flow into their intrinsic energy minima; insofar as energy minima reproduce themselves, they are de facto memories of the system. It follows that there is no one-to-one correspondence between a memory/attractor and the activation of a particular neuron. Instead, a memory corresponds to a pattern of activation and suppression of a very large number of neurons of the network. Learning occurs when the system acquires new attractors or energy minima; this is accomplished by adjusting the synaptic strength between many neurons.

In these networks, memories are *content addressable:* If part of a system enters an activation pattern that matches that of a memory/attractor, the remainder of the system will flow into an activation pattern that "fleshes out" the attractor as a whole. Different portions of the system that code different components of a memory can each be "seeded" with input information that will reproduce the memory in its entirety.

As content-addressable memory systems, these simulations have an intuitive appeal in relationship to actual human memory storage and access. Different small "chunks" of information—a facial profile, the sound of a voice, a name—can recall the memory of a whole person, which includes a myriad of details (e.g., appearance, manner, recollections of past interactions such as conversations). People can identify a particular symphony or rock song on the basis of any one of a number of bars of music. Content-addressable memory in humans is required for tasks ranging from spatial pattern recognition to complex problem solving by matching new problems with old ones whose solutions are known. Mental flexibility is guaranteed by different pathways to the same memory. Artificial neural network systems also demonstrate this flexibility. A specific memory can be "precipitated out" by "seeding" these systems with any one of a number of different portions of the memory.

Information processing is carried out *in parallel;* thus, different modules (smaller networks) compute their outputs simultaneously and check the outputs of other modules so that the overall energy of the larger network is minimized. Information is said to be *distributed* in these systems. In other words, representations are coded by patterns of activation and deactivation across and within neural modules. The overall neural network operates by seeking its minimum energy in response to new input information flowing into the system.

The phenomenology of consciousness briefly described at the beginning of this chapter fits neatly with a neural network–driven hypothesis offered by Rumelhart et al. (1986). They suggest that the content of consciousness is determined by a subset of neurons of the larger system, and that content is expressed (i.e., experienced) when the overall activation pattern of these neurons is relatively stable over a few hundred milliseconds. Our phenomenological reflections suggested that sensory and/or emotive representation are required for conscious experience to emerge—

even abstractions and generalities need to be instantiated with these representations in order to enter this realm. Neural systems subtending these sensory/emotive representations then might correspond to the special subset of neurons proposed by Rumelhart et al. as responsible for conscious experience.

The second principle—namely, that consciousness of something requires a temporally stable brain activation pattern—is implicit in the energy minima concept described above. The overall system, including its subset of "consciousness-determining" elements, will tend to enter temporarily stable states. This tendency is an immediate consequence of the fact that energy minima are functional attractors that stabilize until new inputs shift the neural system into another energy minimum.

## Neurobiological Considerations

Regional cerebral metabolic studies of mental exercises and language processing in nonimpaired subjects have established that activation of multiple diverse cortical areas is required for even simple cognitive tasks (Petersen et al. 1990; Roland 1984). Most importantly for this discussion, many studies indicate that information does not flow unidirectionally from posterior sensory receptive areas to frontal executive and output areas. Instead, simultaneous, bidirectional exchange of information is the rule. Functional reciprocity is anatomically reflected in the fact that projections from posterior association cortex to frontal areas are inevitably accompanied by projections in the opposite direction (Goldman-Rakic 1988; Mesulam 1990). Intracranial recording in humans teaches a similar lesson: neuronal activation in the language output (Broca's) area occurs simultaneously with—not after—neuronal activation in the semantic association (Wernicke's) area during language-production tasks, suggesting reciprocal coupling of these cortical areas (Mesulam 1990). Even *within* posterior cortical regions, reciprocal exchange of information has been observed: von der Heydt et al. (1984) demonstrated backprojections from visual-object–detection microcircuits to primary visual neurons in monkeys. These neurobiological observations support the following hypotheses:

1. Any information-processing task (whether consciously apprehended or not) emerges from the complex, bidirectional interaction of anatomically distributed neural circuits.
2. There is no module that functions as a final arbiter determining the outcomes of these interactions.

These hypotheses are consistent with the findings of neuropsychological studies. In a review paper, Damasio (1989) noted that the destruction of so-called higher-level cortical areas such as frontal and temporal cortex does not block conscious perception. However, damage to certain sensory association areas does impair perceptual representations: "[D]amage in early visual association cortices can disrupt perception of color, texture, stereopsis and spatial placement of the physical components of the stimulus" (Damasio 1989, p. 33). Moreover, these neuropsychological defects are accompanied by parallel impairments in the ability to re-create and recall imagistically these perceptual experiences. Thus, perception and image production are not postulated to be topographically located "downstream" in "higher order" association cortex areas. Instead, in the case of visual perception, association cortical areas are postulated by Damasio to functionally "bind" together lower-order systems coding for visual features through "time-locked retroactivation." Time-locked retroactivation corresponds to reciprocal interaction between cortical regions so that neural modules in sensory areas fire in synchronized patterns. This synchronization process is postulated to cause multiple-feature representations to be organized into a coherent representation of an object. Similarly, representations of objects are postulated to be "bound" together into a representation of an event by association cortex; here, multiple objects are represented in sequence over time. In these models, higher-level processes are facilitative but not sufficient in themselves to yield conscious experience. Conscious experience occurs only when there is a coordinated activation of one or more cortical areas dedicated to sensory representations.

The concepts of "feature binding" and "time-locked" stability of neural modules have received considerable attention and, because they are complex concepts, deserve some special discussion (see also Crick 1994). Time-locked feature binding assumes that different neuronal elements are recruited into a common, resonant, in-phase oscillatory firing pattern whenever inputs are apprehended as a unitary gestalt. Such firing patterns are autocatalytic (i.e., for brief periods they tend to re-create themselves and therefore achieve stability over time). Recruiting additional neurons into a resonant firing process tends to further stabilize this temporal process.

The most striking demonstration of time-locked feature binding was a study by Gray et al. (1989). The responses of visual cortical neurons to light-bar stimulation were studied in the cat. Five to seven neurons in different areas of the visual cortex were recorded simultaneously. Receptive fields of these neurons were nonoverlapping (i.e, a small light stimulus could activate one neuron and not the others). By using independent stimuli, different cells could be coactivated and found to fire according to an oscillatory pattern (Figure 5–1). The temporal relationship of firing patterns across neurons was determined. When light-bar stimuli moved in different directions in different receptive fields, neurons responsive to those receptive fields would activate, but in an uncoordinated fashion. However, when two light-bar stimuli moved in the same direction in two different receptive fields, oscillatory activity of the two corresponding neurons became weakly synchronized over time. Synchronization of oscillatory behavior of different neurons became pronounced when responses were elicited by a single long light bar that covered different receptive fields. "This suggests that (oscillatory) synchronization (of firing patterns of different neurons) depends on global features of the stimuli such as coherent motion and continuity" (Gray et al. 1989, p. 335), which subtend object identification. Feature-binding oscillations were observed to occur in the 40- to 60-Hz range in the Gray et al. study. Roughly similar findings have been reported by Eckhorn et al. (1988).

A series of studies by Freeman and colleagues (for a summary, see Skarda and Freeman 1987) have also underscored the impor-

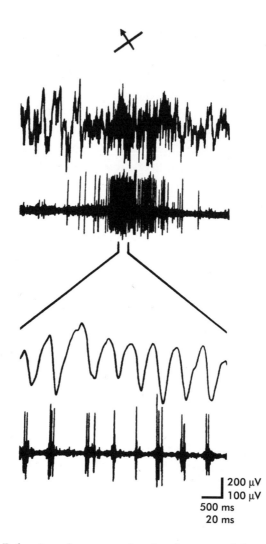

**Figure 5–1.**   Behavior of a neuron in visual cortex of the cat in response to a light bar. The bottom two tracings are enlargements of the top two tracings in time and reflect local field potentials and a single-unit extracellular recording. Note that the single-unit recording reveals a robust oscillatory trend that is in phase with the oscillatory field potential recorded in the neighborhood of that neuron.

*Source.*   Reproduced from Gray CM, Singer W: Stimulus-specific neuronal oscillations in orientation columns of cat visual cortex. *Proc Natl Acad Sci U S A* 86:1699, 1989. Copyright © 1989, C. M. Gray. Used with permission.

tance of temporal coherence of spatially distributed neural processes during perceptual processing. These investigators used a large number of intracortical electroencephalographic (EEG) electrodes to sample electrical activity in the olfactory bulb of the rabbit. The olfactory bulb is not a peripheral nerve but in fact an extension of the central nervous system with a multilayered (albeit primitive) cortical organization. This neural system thus provides an ideal opportunity for direct study of cortical perceptual processing. Rabbits with multielectrode implants were trained to recognize certain smells. It was found that a particular smell induced a particular, synchronous EEG firing pattern distributed across the entire olfactory bulb (as reflected by approximately 60 recording sites). As in the Gray et al. (1989) and Eckhorn et al. (1988) studies, "carrier waves" associated with the detection of a particular olfactory "gestalt" occurred in the 40- to 60-Hz frequency range. However, unlike those in the former studies, the carrier waves discovered by the Skarda/Freeman team expressed not simple sinusoidal oscillations but more complex firing patterns distributed across a wider range of frequencies.

More recent attractor-type neural network computer simulations utilize time-locked oscillatory activation during perceptual gestalt detection (Wang et al. 1990). These simulations enable a precise dissection of the temporal binding that may underlie information processing by biological networks. For instance, these networks deal with perceptual ambiguity in a very interesting fashion. Assume that an input stimulus is presented to the network that can be associated with more than one gestalt stored in memory. The network enters synchronous oscillations involving neurons coding first for one gestalt, then abruptly switches to an oscillatory pattern involving neurons coding for an alternative gestalt (Figure 5–2). These switch processes are reminiscent of the perceptual switches induced when a human subject views a Necker cube (Figure 5–3). We see one facet of the cube first as the forward face and then as the rear face. In general, the gestalt currently held "in mind" by the simulated network is primarily determined not by which subset of neurons is active, but rather by which subset demonstrates temporally coordinated oscillatory firing.

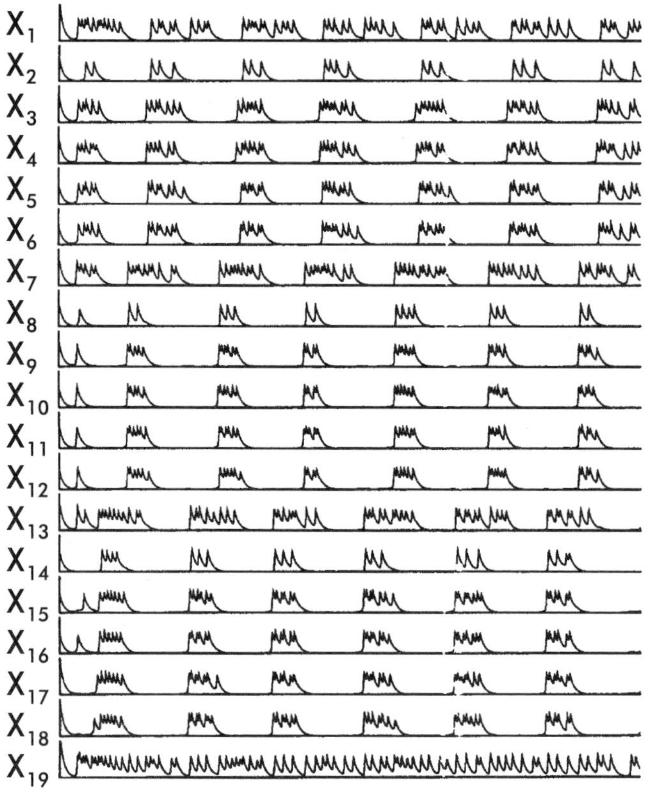

**Figure 5–2.** An artificial network developed by Wang et al. (1990). The behavior of 19 neurons that have been simultaneously activated by stimulation external to the network is shown. The $y$ axis corresponds to the firing rate, and the $x$ axis represents time. Neurons 1–6 code for one memory; neurons 7–12, for a second memory; and neurons 13–18, for a third memory. Because all neurons are activated equally, the system cannot decide which memory is the "best fit" with respect to input information. Consequently, the network rapidly shifts between representations of each of the three memories. When the system is "in" a particular memory, oscillatory firing of neurons coding for that memory is synchronous. The critical insight provided by these networks is that information is coded not only by a distributed pattern of oscillatory activation but also by whether that activation is in phase, or "time locked."

*Source.*   Reproduced from Wang D, Buhmann J, von der Malsburg C: Pattern segmentation in associative memory. *Neural Computation* 2:102, 1990. Copyright © 1990, MIT Press. Used with permission.

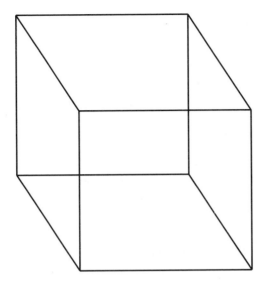

**Figure 5–3.** A Necker cube. When viewing this stimulus, human observers will alternate between two different perspectives at a relatively rapid rate. This perceptual switch process is reminiscent of that demonstrated by the artificial neural network in Figure 5–2 in response to an ambiguous stimulus that has multiple "interpretations."

## Toward a Theory of Conscious Experience

This discussion suggests the following hypothesis:

> Forty- to 60-Hz time-locked oscillatory neural firing not only "binds" features across different neural areas to create gestalts but itself constitutes the neural correlate of conscious experience.

This is not an original hypothesis; a similar proposal has also been described in a recent book by Francis Crick (1994) and a review paper by Baringa (1989). As discussed earlier, I propose that neural systems responsible for sensory and/or emotive encoding are captured by these oscillatory processes; if time-locked oscillatory activation incorporates a critical mass of neurons from these modules over a critical period of time, then a conscious experience will hypothetically emerge.

If this model has validity, neurobiological processes responsible for conscious experience are likely to be self-perpetuating: resonant oscillatory processes tend to sustain themselves. Conscious experience would therefore be an indicator of stability and retention of activated representations at a cortical level. I have also proposed that resonant, oscillatory processes tend to recruit additional neural network components into this synchronous process (which further sustain the representational state). Therefore, a second neurobiological consequence of a conscious state would be the functional *integration* of different cortical modules; a similar proposal also has been made by Baars (1983). However, my position is that it is not conscious experience itself that is doing the integrating; rather, conscious experience is the indicator that such integration is occurring at a neurobiological level.

## Limitations of the Model

Our conscious experience is extremely sensitive to change. Indeed, it is entirely plausible that in the absence of perceptual change or contrast, an object of consciousness would drift out of awareness (Wittgenstein 1980a). If all we saw was red, we would orient to nothing. A red square on a white background, on the other hand, provides a perceptual contrast that we can attentionally revisit periodically to remind ourselves of the squareness in our visual field. A sound in the background becomes far more noticeable when its pitch changes. A pressure on one's arm becomes much more noticeable when the pressure, tactilely speaking, moves. The major exception to this rule is emotion—we can persistently experience anxiety or sadness, for instance, over a period of hours to days and even longer, without habituating to the experience.

I have proposed that consciousness requires stable, synchronous activation distributed across sensory/somatic representational modules. Contrast or change—the phenomenological edge that reawakens consciousness—would seem to destroy stability of synchronous activation of neuronal systems.

The change/contrast dependence of conscious experience represents a serious challenge to our model, but recently developed neural network simulations actually predict the importance of these factors. For instance, a network developed by Hjelmfelt and Ross (1994) uses simulated neurons that are much more "biological" than are standard attractor networks; they obey standard physiological equations for excitable membranes. Inputs to these systems also cause them to settle into attractors that are coded by synchronous oscillatory activity. However, these states are only transient; a Hjelmfelt/Ross network will soon drift back to a neutral "at rest" attractor. (It is noteworthy that an "at rest" attractor was also characterized physiologically for the olfactory system of rabbits by Skarda and Freeman [1987].) These artificial networks will therefore maintain states distinct from the "at rest" state only if stimulus configurations are altered at fairly frequent intervals. Thus, the model demonstrates stable synchrony across groups of neurons—but only on a temporary basis—unless restimulated with new configurations of inputs. The experiential persistence of emotion relative to sensory images remains a mystery and may reflect fundamental differences in neural circuitry relative to sensory systems.

Conscious experience in a conventional sense does not occur unless the content of consciousness is somehow remembered, even if temporarily. A limitation of the model is that the mnemonic aspect of conscious experience is not captured explicitly. There has been much research—and speculation—about how neurobiological systems store new information, including memory traces of their own prior states. The hippocampus is a relatively small region of the limbic system that nonetheless has diverse reciprocal connections with multiple cortical areas, including sensory representational regions for visual and auditory processing. These connections seem to play an essential role in the gestation of memories (Rolls 1990); current thinking is that the hippocampus coordinates the storage of memories in distributed cortical systems (Mesulam 1990). Therefore, a prediction of this model of conscious experience is that distributed, synchronous activation of neural systems is necessary in order for storage of information to be coordinated by the hippocampus. In terms of oscillatory attractor models of neural information processing, this outcome would correspond to shifts in interneuron connectivity that facilitate resonant activation corresponding to the prior conscious experience. A version of the experience then becomes reaccessible through future neural information processing. I am not aware of research data supporting this view (or contradicting it), but it is hard to imagine a mechanism of conscious experience that does not also lead directly to storage of some neural representation of that experience in memory so that it can be recalled at a later time.

Of course, the relationship between memory and conscious experience also works in the opposite direction. Much conscious experience consists of memories—ranging from recollections of events in the past to complex learned knowledge. The model that I propose therefore assumes that the recollection of previously stored memories, if experienced consciously, also activates sensory or emotive modules in a time-locked, synchronous fashion.

## Toward a Theory of Unconscious Mental Processes

What does this model of consciousness provide as hypotheses regarding unconscious mental processes?

**First,** the model suggests that most brain processes are unconscious. In particular, information processing by cortical (and subcortical) modules not directly responsible for sensory or emotive encoding will remain outside of consciousness if these brain events do not, in turn, result in activation of sensory/emotive modules. Neurons in the frontal cortex, cerebellum, or striatum, even if firing in a totally coordinated fashion, probably do not yield particular conscious experience even though their information-processing capacities are critical for intelligent, purposeful behavior.

**Second,** the model suggests that conscious mental processes do not "control" unconscious processes (see also Dennett 1991). Instead, consciousness might be better conceptualized as a kind of episodic readout of ongoing unconscious neural computation that is projected onto the screen(s) of our sensory/emotive representational systems. This is not to say that neural correlates of conscious experience cannot influence brain processes. Modules responsible for coding conscious experience would, in theory, freely interact with other neural modules, which would lead to new conscious experiences as well as unconscious information-processing and motoric actions (e.g., speech, limb movements). For example, I could say inwardly to myself the phrase "I want an apple" and follow this by later walking to the kitchen, opening the refrigerator door, and grabbing an apple. However, cortical circuits influenced by a biological need for nutrition and responsible for stored knowledge about sources of nutrition such as apples, the remembrance that I purchased apples yesterday, the knowledge that the apples are located in the kitchen, and so forth, were also active—more or less unconsciously—and all collectively interact so that the bit of inner speech that stated, "I want an apple" and the ensuing behaviors result. Conscious experience therefore has the appearance of punctuations of otherwise unconscious neural processes blending input, stored information, and output that express momentary resonant stability of particular activated neural modules. Instead of a controlling agent "within the brain"—that is, a homunculus directing information processing and equated with consciousness—the model predicts that the "controller" is an emergent property arising from the blend of input, output, and stored neural information unfolding over time. The brain contains only neurons, and no neuron or set of neurons (including those neurons subtending conscious experience) is prepotent. The absence of an executive agency may be philosophically offensive to some people, but it is difficult to draw any other conclusion from our current knowledge of brain function and neural networks.

**Third,** the model predicts that neurobiological systems responsible for sensory and emotive representations can be active but *not* be registered consciously. In theory, at least four types of neuronal activation involving these systems would not be conscious:

1. *Activation of a critical mass of neuronal elements has not been achieved.* Presumably, only two cooperatively firing neurons in sensory areas will not result in a conscious experience. A critical

mass of neurons in appropriate areas must be cooperatively activated. The amount of neuronal coordination that leads to a conscious experience may be quite variable and dependent on the modality of that experience. Emotion coding may require only a few hundred neurons in subcortical centers, whereas complex linguistic representations probably involves coordinated activation of many millions of neurons.

2. *Oscillatory processes occur outside some critical frequency range.* I have proposed that the critical frequency range of oscillatory neural activation is 40–70 Hz. A common example of an oscillatory process occurring outside this range is the alpha rhythm. Activation of cortical modules via an alpha rhythm (frequency range of 8–12 Hz) fails to produce conscious experience. There is some evidence, for instance, that the alpha rhythm actually increases the conscious stimulus detection threshold (Bohdanecky et al. 1984). However, oscillatory activation occurring outside the 40- to 70-Hz range could theoretically result in significant information processing (while remaining outside of conscious awareness).

3. *Oscillatory processes are not sustained for a critical period of time.* I have proposed that resonant oscillatory activation needs to be sustained for a few hundred milliseconds in order for a conscious experience to emerge. Such activation for shorter periods of time could also result in significant information processing but remain outside of consciousness. Critical duration thresholds for oscillatory synchrony emerging as conscious experience are likely to be quite variable. Perhaps detection of more complex representations (e.g., linguistic) requires stable oscillatory firing for many hundreds of milliseconds, whereas detection of a simple flash of light requires synchronous firing that lasts only tens of milliseconds. Different aspects of the same experience—for instance, becoming conscious of "what" I am seeing versus "where" I am seeing, or detecting sounds versus detecting the meaning of those sounds as speech— may require different time durations for neural representation (for a suggestive perceptual study, see Atkinson and Braddick 1989).

4. *Oscillatory processes are not synchronized.* Our model suggests that activation of sensory/emotive modules, even if sustained in the appropriate frequency range for a sufficient duration, will not produce a conscious experience unless oscillatory synchronization across neural groups has occurred.

A now-classic demonstration of unconscious activation of sensory cortical modules is "blindsight." "Blindsight" refers to residual capacities of patients with damage to the visual cortex. These patients are tested by presenting visual stimuli specifically to their blinded visual fields. They report "seeing" nothing but nonetheless are often able to correctly "guess" which object is present in their blind visual field (Weiskrantz 1986). Our simple model suggests a wide range of nonconscious neural processing that could account for blindsight—all that is required is that time-locked, oscillatory activation of sensory/emotive coding regions of sufficient extent and duration does *not* occur. Nothing in our theory specifies that meaningful information processing *requires* time-locked, oscillatory synchronization.

A specific consequence of this approach is that the same type of sensory or emotive activation under different circumstances may at times lead to conscious awareness and at other times remain outside of the range of consciousness. For instance, if a stimulus is expected, less meaningful or sustained input may still induce coherent oscillatory activation of a critical mass of neurons (cf. Dietrich and Theios 1992). Conversely, stimulation in peripheral versus foveal visual fields is unlikely to have the same efficacy in mobilizing visual sensory representational neurons.

An additional consequence of this model is that memories could be activated while still remaining outside of the realm of conscious experience; this would occur when activation did not directly engage sensory or emotive systems or engaged them in a nonsynchronous fashion. A "Freudian" unconscious—wherein certain memories are expressed, but only indirectly through symptoms or actions rather than via conscious recollection—is entirely consistent with the model of conscious experience described above.

My comments regarding the necessary instability of input information in order to enter into consciousness suggest pathways into information processing that can remain outside of conscious awareness. For instance, inputs that are very constant may have great information-processing significance yet fall outside of awareness. A pilot cannot be continually aware that the sky is blue but must immediately be attentive to where the blue ends and the horizon begins. We generally cease to be attentive to the clothes that we are wearing soon after we put them on.

This perspective may also account for hypnotic phenomena induced by staring at an object or a swinging pendulum. These exercises produce an unchanging stimulus or stimulus pattern which in turn mutes conscious awareness of the object itself (as well as other external stimuli). So-called autohypnotic or dissociative states associated with previous traumatic experiences could be similarly accounted for—the persistent, intrusive reexperiencing of memories of the trauma could produce an unchanging pattern of internally generated stimuli that also curtail conscious awareness.

My discussion would not be complete if the implications of the model in terms of other sorts of psychopathology were not considered. I have already provided one such example: an inability to refrain from recalling certain traumatic memories that persist in reappearing in consciousness. However, a host of other syndromes exist in which particular representational elements repetitively force themselves into consciousness. Examples include delusions of the *idée fixe* type (wherein the affected patient is preoccupied, for example, with the possibility that the CIA is operating behind his back or that his wife is cheating on him). Patients with obsessive-compulsive disorder experience repeated intrusions into conscious awareness of images and emotions associated with dirt, disease, bodily harm, or catastrophe. Certain affective disorders, such as depression, may be associated with the reexperiencing of "depressogenic" memories in the present. Perhaps new neurobiological treatments for these disorders—yet to be discovered—can be developed by uncoupling resonant cortical modules, forcing cortical activation out a critical power-spectrum range, or shortening the duration of resonant neural processes essential for these pathogenic neural representations. Disrupting these representations may have the added benefit of preventing their registration and storage in memory. Reliving memories of delusions, obsessions, and traumatic events is likely to reinforce their pathological effects. Breaking this vicious cycle could therefore have therapeutic effects.

## Concluding Remarks

It must be stressed that empirical evidence supporting this model is sparse, and it will surely be replaced by more sophisticated approaches based on emerging neurobiological and computer simulation findings. Nonetheless, reviews of early research in this area reveal that the importance of coactivation of multiple systems has been appreciated for some time. Evidence, although preliminary, suggests that different neural modules become functionally coupled only if their activation patterns oscillate in a synchronized fashion. Extrapolating from these findings, one can propose a vehicle for higher forms of complex mentation. It may be that only particular types of coordinated activity result in conscious experience. What enters into consciousness would then reflect only the tip of an iceberg of coordinated neural activity. Attempting to specify necessary neural-processing conditions for emergence of conscious experience only highlights the vastness of neural processing that remains outside of human awareness. Improved delineation of the neurobiological boundary between conscious and unconscious mental processes may provide important clues to the mechanisms and possible treatments of a range of psychiatric syndromes.

## References

Amit DJ: Modeling Brain Function: The World of Attractor Neural Networks. Cambridge, UK, Cambridge University Press, 1989

Atkinson J, Braddick OJ: "Where" and "what" in visual search. Perception 18:181–189, 1989

Baars BJ: Conscious contents provide the nervous system with coherent, global information, in Consciousness and Self-Regulation, Vol 3. Edited by Davidson RJ, Schwartz GE, Shapiro D. New York, Plenum, 1983, pp 41–79

Baringa M: The mind revealed? Science 249:856–858, 1989

Bohdanecky Z, Bozkov V, Radil T: Acoustic stimulus threshold related to EEG alpha and non-alpha epochs. Int J Psychophysiol 2:63–66, 1984

Churchland PS, Sejnowski TJ: Perspectives on cognitive neuroscience. Science 242:741–745, 1988

Crick F: The Astonishing Hypothesis: The Scientific Search for the Soul. New York, Charles Scribner's Sons, 1994

Damasio AR: Time-locked multiregional retroactivation: a systems-level proposal for the neural substrates of recall and recognition. Cognition 33:25–62, 1989

Dennett DC: Consciousness Explained. Boston, MA, Little, Brown, 1991

Dietrich D, Theios J: Priming outside of awareness and subsequent stimulus identification. Percept Mot Skills 75:483–497, 1992

Eckhorn R, Bauer R, Jordan W, et al: Coherent oscillations: a mechanism of feature linking in the visual cortex? Biol Cybern 60:121–130, 1988

Gelernter D: The Muse in the Machine. New York, Free Press, 1994

Gevins AS, Morgan NH, Bressler SL, et al: Human neuroelectric patterns predict performance activity. Science 235:580–585, 1987

Goldman-Rakic P: Changing concepts of cortical connectivity: parallel distributed cortical networks. Ann Rev Neurosci 11:137–156, 1988

Gray CM, Singer W: Stimulus-specific neuronal oscillations in orientation columns of cat visual cortex. Proc Natl Acad Sci U S A 86:1698–1702, 1989

Gray CM, König P, Engel AK, et al: Oscillatory responses in cat visual cortex exhibit inter-columnar synchronization which reflects global stimulus properties. Nature 338:334–337, 1989

Hinton GE, Shallice T: Lesioning an attractor network: investigations of acquired dyslexia. Psychol Rev 98:74–95, 1991

Hjelmfelt A, Ross J: Pattern recognition, chaos and multiplicity in neural networks of excitable systems. Proc Natl Acad Sci U S A 91:63–67, 1994

Hoffman RE: Computer simulations of neural information processing and the schizophrenia–mania dichotomy. Arch Gen Psychiatry 44:178–187, 1987

Hoffman RE, Kravitz RE: Feedforward action regulation and the experience of will. Behavioral and Brain Sciences 10:782–783, 1987

Hopfield JJ: Neural networks and physical systems with emergent collective computational abilities. Proc Natl Acad Sci U S A 79:2554–2558, 1982

Jenkins WM, Merzenich MM, Ochs MT, et al: Functional reorganization of the primary somatosensory cortex in adult owl monkeys after behaviorally controlled tactile stimulation. J Neurophysiol 63:82–104, 1990

Mesulam M-M: Large-scale neurocognitive networks and distributed processing for attention, language and memory. Ann Neurol 28:597–613, 1990

Montgomery EB, Clare MH, Sahrmann S, et al: Neuronal multipotentiality: evidence for network representation of physiological function. Brain Res 580:49–61, 1992

Papanicolaou AC: Emotion: A Reconsideration of the Somatic Theory. New York, Gordon & Breach, 1989

Petersen SE, Fox PT, Synder AZ, et al: Activation of extrastriate and frontal cortical areas by visual words and word-like stimuli. Science 249:1041–1044, 1990

Roland PE: Metabolic measurements of the working frontal cortex in man. Trends Neurosci 7:430–435, 1984

Rolls ET: Functions of neuronal networks in the hippocampus and back-projections in the cerebral cortex in memory, in Brain Organization and Memory: Cells, Systems, and Circuits. Edited by McGaugh JL, Lynch G. New York, Oxford University Press, 1990

Rumelhart DE, Smolensky P, McClelland JL, et al: Schemata and sequential thought processes in PDP models, in Parallel Distributed Processing: Explorations in the Microstructure of Cognition, Vol 2. Edited by McClelland JL, Rumelhart DE, PDP Research Group. Cambridge, MA, MIT Press, 1986, pp 7–57

Skarda CA, Freeman WJ: How brains make chaos in order to make sense of the world. Behavioral and Brain Sciences 10:161–195, 1987

Smolensky P: Information processing in dynamical systems: foundations of Harmony Theory, in Parallel Distributed Processing: Explorations in the Microstructure of Cognition, Vol 1: Foundations. Edited by Rumelhart DE, McClelland JL, PDP Research Group. Cambridge, MA, MIT Press, 1986, pp 194–281

von der Heydt R, Peterhans E, Baumgartner G: Illusory contours and cortical neuron responses. Science 224:1260–1262, 1984

Wang D, Buhmann J, von der Malsburg C: Pattern segmentation in associative memory. Neural Computation 2:94–106, 1990

Weiskrantz L: Blindsight: A Case Study and Implications. Oxford, UK, Clarendon Press, 1986

Wittgenstein L: Remarks on the Philosophy of Psychology, Vol 1. Edited by Anscombe GEM, von Wright GH. Chicago, IL, University of Chicago Press, 1980a

Wittgenstein L: Remarks on the Philosophy of Psychology, Vol 2. Edited by von Wright GH, Nyman H. Chicago, IL, University of Chicago Press, 1980b

# Chapter 6

# *Rethinking Repression*

Dan J. Stein, M.B., and Jeffrey E. Young, Ph.D.

I n psychoanalytic formulations of the unconscious, repression is an extremely important notion, the "corner-stone on which the whole structure of psychoanalysis rests" (Freud 1915/1957, p. 16). Components of this hypothesis of repression include the notions that 1) painful ideas are defended against 2) by being pushed into an unconscious realm, 3) where they continue to exert influence, 4) perhaps resulting in symptoms. These concepts are central to the Freudian view of mind and of psychopathology.

Although long neglected by mainstream academic psychology, repression has been an important topic of experimental investigation for many years. For example, during the 1930s and 1940s, experimenters tried to provide evidence for repression by using various laboratory paradigms such as differential recall of pleasant and unpleasant memories. Since the cognitive revolution (see Chapter 1 in this volume), empirical study of unconscious processes including repression has been a growing area of study (Erdelyi 1985; Singer 1990).

Whether or not repression will remain an important construct for the new integrative study of the cognitive unconscious is somewhat unclear. Erdelyi (1990), for example, has claimed that Freud added an important dimension—the defensive dimension—to our understanding of the operation of schemas in the mind. Singer and Sincoff (1990), on the other hand, have emphasized that individuals differ in the cognitive-affective strategies they use; these authors have begun to move away from using the term *repression.* In this chapter, we attempt to reframe the psychodynamic theory of repression in a way that is consistent with developments in contemporary cognitive science.

# Psychoanalysis

As is true for many of the central terms of psychoanalysis, the notion of repression has been used in various ways, both in the writings of Freud and in subsequent work. It is useful to begin by considering this developmental history. Fortunately, Erdelyi and colleagues (Erdelyi 1985; Erdelyi and Goldberg 1979) have provided a detailed exegesis from which we will draw liberally.

Freud's first description of the process of repression is found in an early formulation of his conflict theory of hysteria (Freud 1892–1893/1966), at a time preceding the discovery of psychoanalysis. His theory evolved in the context of treating a woman who presented with symptoms of poor lactation and vomiting during breast feeding. Freud hypothesized an underlying ambivalence about the breast feeding, a conflict of which the patient was not aware. The patient dealt with the distressing idea (i.e., her disinclination to breast feed) by inhibiting it. As Freud postulated, "the distressing antithetical idea, which has the appearance of being inhibited, is removed from association with the intention and continues to exist as a disconnected idea, often unconsciously to the patient" (1892–1893/1966, p. 122). He noted, however, that this idea could "put itself into effect through the agencies of the somatic innervations" (p. 122), thus resulting in symptoms.

Freud's first use of the term repression followed soon afterward in his "Preliminary Communication" with Breuer (Breuer and Freud 1893/1955), which later became the first section of "Studies on Hysteria." At this point, he used the terms *repression, suppression, inhibition,* and *dissociation* interchangeably, writing that "it is a question which the patient wished to forget, and therefore intentionally repressed from his conscious thought and inhibited and suppressed" (Breuer and Freud 1893/1955, p. 10). In "Studies on Hysteria" (Breuer and Freud 1893–1895/1955), repression continues to be given a central place in the pathogenesis of hysteria.

Repression may involve inhibition of either an idea or an affect. In 1894, Freud wrote that a painful idea could be dealt with by repressing its emotional content: " . . . defense against the incompatible idea was effected by separating it from its affect; the idea itself remained in consciousness" (Freud 1894/1962, p. 58). This phenomenon was later termed *isolation*. Thus, from early on, Freud differentiated obsessional and hysterical patients—the hysterical patient repressed ideas, whereas the obsessional patient repressed affect.

In 1915, in an article entitled "Repression," Freud wrote that "the essence of repression lies simply in the function of turning something away and keeping it at a distance from consciousness" (Freud 1915/1957, p. 147). Erdelyi (1985) emphasized that this definition of repression does not specify whether repression is conscious or unconscious. What is, however, central to Freud's construct is the notion of motivated inhibition—repression attempts to reduce or prevent some form of psychological pain.

In "Inhibitions, Symptoms and Anxiety," Freud (1926/1959) attempted to differentiate *repression* and *defense*, describing repression as a specific type of defense, one that involves direct inhibition of a thought, impulse, or memory. Nevertheless, Freud continued to use the notion of repression in the broadest sense. As Erdelyi and Goldberg (1979) have pointed out, this inconsistency is explained by the fact that all defense mechanisms involve repression in some sense; the narrow sense of repression is used only to express a variant of the more general notion.

The importance of Freud's theory of repression is difficult to overestimate. He expertly described a range of clinical phenomena, and his theory of the unconscious mind provides a powerful model for understanding the pathogenesis of these phenomena and for deriving suitable means for intervention. Nevertheless, it is important to go beyond this pioneering work. In particular, Freud's notion of repression is based, like the rest of his work, on the outdated metapsychology of psychic energetics. There is little contemporary support for this theoretical underpinning (Rosenblatt and Thickstun 1977; Swanson 1977), so that the question arises of how to reconceptualize Freud's observations.

Within psychoanalysis there have in fact been a number of attempts to reframe theory in more cognitive terms (Stein, Chapter 1 in this volume). Freud's own theory of signal anxiety is reminiscent of later cybernetic constructs. Furthermore, since Freud's

work, a number of psychoanalysts have conceptualized unconscious processes in terms of rule-based operations (Eagle 1987).
Suppes and Warren (1975) for example, defined defense mechanisms as transformations of propositions: "By a transformation we
mean a function that maps unconscious propositions (thoughts
or impulses) into conscious propositions; a transformation may
also be thought of as a process that takes unconscious propositions
and changes them in specific ways into conscious propositions"
(pp. 405–406). This kind of theorizing leads immediately to work
done in cognitive psychology.

## Cognitive Psychology

Although psychodynamic theory has long fallen outside the mainstream of academic psychology, there has always been some interest in and awareness of its constructs (Dollard and Miller 1950).
Even in the early decades of this century, there was a great deal of
empirical investigation that attempted to verify psychodynamic
theory in general and the notion of repression in particular (Jung
1906/1918; Rapaport 1942). In a more recent and rather skeptical
review, Holmes (1990) enumerated five approaches to the experimental study of repression.

**First**, since the 1930s, differential recall of pleasant and unpleasant experiences has been examined in several laboratories. It
might be hypothesized that pleasant memories are more readily
recalled, whereas unpleasant memories are repressed. Nevertheless, a number of contradictory findings, including the demonstration that both markedly unpleasant and pleasant memories are
more easily recalled than are more neutral ones. The relevance of
this body of research to the theory of repression is, however,
questionable (Rapaport 1942). As Erdelyi and Goldberg (1979)
have pointed out, not all unpleasant memories are repressed.

**Second,** another area of study has been differential recall of
completed and uncompleted tasks. The Zeigarnik effect (Zeigarnik 1927) states that completed tasks are better recalled. In
several experiments, it was found that fewer uncompleted than
completed tasks were remembered under conditions of higher

stress (i.e., when tasks were presented as intelligence tests) than of lower stress (i.e., when no importance was attached to the tasks). A number of criticisms have been leveled at this research, including the argument that decreased recall in this paradigm may be a result of differential learning (Holmes 1990).

**Third**, changes in recall have been associated with the introduction and elimination of stress. In this paradigm, experimental and control subjects are tested for ability to recall neutral stimuli. After subjects have been exposed to stress associated with this task (e.g., through failure of a test involving the learned materials), recall is tested again. Finally, stress is eliminated (e.g., through good performance on a test involving the materials) and recall tested one last time. In many cases, subjects' recall was found to diminish after stress induction and to increase after stress elimination ("return of the repressed"). Holmes (1990) has argued, however, that far from demonstrating the existence of repression, such results merely reflect the interference of stress.

**Fourth**, several researchers have investigated individual differences in repression. One approach involves the use of the Repression-Sensitization Scale (Byrne et al. 1963), which is composed of items from the Minnesota Multiphasic Personality Inventory that ask about the presence of various symptoms. Subjects with low scores are termed "repressors," and those with high scores are termed "sensitizers." Holmes (1990) has pointed out that this differentiation says nothing about the psychoanalytic concept of repression per se. In another approach, a number of researchers have found correlations between a need for achievement and increased recall of uncompleted versus completed tasks. However, this finding contradicts what might have been expected by a psychoanalytic theory of repression. A third research approach (Davis and Schwartz 1987) has defined "repressors" as subjects with high scores on the Marlowe-Crowne Social Desirability Scale and low scores on the Taylor Manifest Anxiety Scale. Such individuals have been found less likely to report stressful or unpleasant events. Again, the question arises of whether these persons are actually unaware of these events or are simply less willing to report them (Holmes 1990).

**Fifth,** yet another area of research has examined perceptual defense (Dixon 1971, 1981; Erdelyi 1974, 1985; Eriksen and Pierce 1968; Holender 1986; Merikle 1982). Early research compared perception of stressful and nonstressful material, showing, for example, that stressful words require a longer exposure time than nonstressful words in order to be read. More recent experiments have used increasingly sophisticated paradigms with subliminal stimuli (Bornstein and Pittman 1992), and have clearly demonstrated the existence of perception outside of awareness. Nevertheless, as Erdelyi (1985) and Shevrin (1990) have conceded, although particular components of the psychoanalytic theory of repression have been demonstrated in the laboratory, no experiment has demonstrated their conjoint activity.

All of these laboratory areas of research, then, provide only indirect forms of evidence for repression in comparison with the direct evidence obtained in clinical work (Cloitre, Chapter 3 in this volume). The failure to reproduce clinical phenomena in the laboratory does not itself imply the nonexistence of such phenomena. Ultimately, more complex forms of empirical research, perhaps combining the videotaping of clinical sessions with cognitive methods (Horowitz et al. 1990), may be necessary if the phenomena of clinical work are to be studied in the laboratory.

In addition to empirical research, there is the question of how best to formulate repression in terms of cognitive psychology theory. A number of early cognitive theorists attempted to formulate defense mechanisms in terms of rule-based operations in a way similar to that proposed by some psychodynamic theorists. Erdelyi (1990), for example, approvingly referenced Suppes and Warren's (1975) conclusion that standard defense mechanisms can be conceptualized as simple transformations.

Some cognitivists have attempted to translate such rule-based theories into the constructs of artificial intelligence. Wegman (1985), for example, suggested that early Freudian notions of repression could be reformulated in terms of script theory. Colby and colleagues (Faught et al. 1977) have in fact simulated defensive transformations in a computational model called PARRY. Consider, for example, the following rule that PARRY uses: "If shame crosses a threshold for paranoia (SHAME equal to 10), the paranoid mode is activated. The first consequence of the paranoid mode is the rejection of the belief that led to the increase in shame by resetting the truth value of the belief . . . . Instead an alternate belief is inferred" (Faught et al. 1977, pp. 175–176).

Freud himself was not greatly impressed by early empirical attempts to validate psychoanalytic constructs (MacKinnon and Dukes 1964). Although the rules of information processing are no longer based on physical laws, they still appear to assume the classical insistence on formal algorithms, with a neglect of meaning and context. Laboratory experimentation has often taken the Helmholtzian route of focusing on neutral stimuli in groups of normal subjects. There has been a relative lack of focus on individual subjects—on the embodiment of mental structures and processes in a specific person's brain in a particular context.

## Embodied Cognition

We are left, then, with the question of how to reformulate psychoanalytic observations in cognitive terms that go beyond energic metapsychology yet retain the clinical concern with the embodiment of cognitive structures and processes in the brain and in social context. In order to proceed, it may be worthwhile to draw a distinction between those cognitivists who have emphasized symbolic cognition and those who have emphasized situated cognition. This division within cognitive science has recently been discussed in depth (Norman 1993).

The characterization presented here of these contrasting positions is intended to be heuristic rather than comprehensive, and may not cover the work of any particular cognitive scientist. The symbolic stance holds that mental activity can be fully described in terms of the processing of symbols, that the underlying physical substrate of this processing mechanism is irrelevant, and that the context of the processing can be explicated fully in terms of the individual's symbol processing. In contrast, the situated position could be said to emphasize the embodiment of mental processes, both in the brain and in a particular interactive context.

There are a number of arguments in favor of an approach that focuses on embodied cognition (Stein, in press). A full account is unfortunately beyond the scope of this book. Lakoff (1987, Chapter 4 in this volume), however, has provided one of the strongest arguments, beginning from an exploration of the way in which humans classify. In opposition to the classical position that categories can be defined formally in terms of necessary and sufficient characteristics (which can be then be referred to in terms of abstract symbols), Lakoff has argued that classification relies on human experience (and therefore reflects the embodiment of mind in brain and in social context).

This kind of stance will not be unfamiliar to clinicians. For example, a concept of embodied cognition is reminiscent of Piaget's account of abstract thought as a phenomenon that can be understood as emerging from the interaction of brain-based schemas with the environment (Piaget 1952). Embodied cognition also brings to mind more recent work on neural networks that shows how abstract symbolic thought emerges from the interaction of simulated neural elements with external stimuli (McClelland et al. 1986; Rumelhart et al. 1986). Finally, from the viewpoint of integrative clinical (including psychoanalytic) work that incorporates biological and sociological factors, embodiment of cognitive processes in the brain and in social interaction seems clear.

Lakoff (1987, Chapter 4 in this volume) also provides a methodology for exploring embodied cognitive structures. Consider, for example, his work on the structure of anger. Whereas the symbolic stance has tended to ignore emotion (or to reduce emotion to the prioritized interruption of different processes by one another [Simon 1967; Sloman 1987]), Lakoff has focused on the metaphors we use to describe anger. He notes, for example, that we talk about ANGER as HEAT. For example, we speak of getting **"hot** under the collar," having a **"heated** argument," "seeing **red,"** and so on. This metaphor is used in a typical scenario in which an offending event produces anger, an attempt is made to control the anger (to "cool off"), but sometimes control is lost (the person "blows up") and an act of retribution occurs. Lakoff argues that this metaphoric mapping reflects human experience of anger, both as a phenomenon with particular psychosomatic correlates (e.g., anger is associated with activation of the autonomic nervous system) and as a phenomenon that emerges in social interaction (e.g., anger is triggered by certain kinds of provocations and results in certain kinds of reactions).

Similarly, in exploring notions of repression, it may be valuable to consider the metaphors of repression in more detail. It is highly likely that such metaphors antedated Freud's writings (Ellenberger 1970). Freud's genius lies in his having translated these commonsense metaphors into a scientific account (cf. Wollheim 1993). What exactly are the metaphors of the mind that are used to describe repression? We would suggest that these typically have to do with the metaphor of MIND as CONTAINER.

## The MIND as CONTAINER Metaphor

Consider the case of a woman who is raped on her way home from work. In the aftermath of this traumatic experience, she finds herself taking a different route home. She does not, however, articulate this change in route until a therapist points out to her that she is avoiding all kinds of stimuli that might remind her of the rape. At this point, she suddenly understands that she has changed her route and why she has changed it. She answers, "You are right. I have pushed the rape to the bottom of my mind. I don't want to think about it."

This patient is using a metaphor of the mind as a container with superficial and deep partitions. Within this container, there are objects—that is, thoughts and feelings—that can move around. Thoughts and feelings at the bottom of the container (where they are out of awareness) come into the top partition (where they are in awareness), but can be pushed back down again. There are a number of expressions that she might have used to refer to this metaphor—"the thought came up," "my feeling surfaced," "I pushed the impulse down," and so forth—all of which reflect the general structure of the metaphor.

One aspect of this metaphor is that the person whose mind is a container is able to act in various ways on the objects (thoughts and feelings) within the container. We have already noted that the objects can be "pushed down." In addition, thoughts can be separated from feelings (e.g., they can go into different partitions). The woman might say, for example, that whenever she traverses her old route, she starts to have palpitations. When the therapist makes the observation that she may be experiencing anxiety, she might say—"You are right. The feeling is what I had during the rape. But although that anxiety keeps coming up, I manage to keep the thought of the rape down."

It would be a mistake to think that these mappings are simply drawn from Freud's topology of the mind. Certainly, Freud's views are now commonplace. But this metaphor has much stronger appeal than do the particulars of Freud's theory. Consider, for example, the response of a subject to some typical instructions from a hypnotist (Hammond 1992). The hypnotist might tell the subject that there are two parts to the mind—a conscious and an unconscious. The hypnotist will talk primarily with the unconscious mind. The subject is to relax, and the unconscious mind will take over and let the hypnotist know when it is ready to go on by raising a finger. Most subjects will understand this metaphor, and some will comply completely with the suggestions of the hypnotist. Such compliance is by no means dependent on the subject's familiarity with psychodynamic theory; rather, the subject is simply making use of a well-known metaphor of the mind. Similarly, the notion that our minds are able to divorce passion from reason was in no way invented by Freud; rather, it involves a metaphor of the mind that has long been central to Western thought.

Certainly, Freud's theory has added to the richness and depth of the folk metaphor. He provided a detailed account of the phenomenology and topology of the partitions and of their workings in terms of the laws of physics, and he focused on how that which is hidden continues to exert an important influence. Freud also devised a detailed explanation of the different kinds of psychopathology (obsessional versus hysterical) based on repression of affect and of ideas, respectively. Freud's elaboration of the folk metaphor is thus an important scientific contribution.

The accuracy of the folk metaphor should not, however, be underestimated. The MIND as CONTAINER metaphor reflects human experience of thoughts and feelings moving in and out of awareness and of our ability to control these thoughts and feelings in various ways. The folk metaphor, and its Freudian elaboration, go beyond some simplistic cognitive views insofar as they tackle the double embodiment of human cognition (i.e., in the brain and in social interaction).

On the other hand, it is obvious that the mind is not really a container. Too literal an acceptance of this metaphor will lead to mistakes. For example, in the Freudian elaboration of the container metaphor, particular repressed memories remain unchanged, waiting to return to consciousness. This view contrasts with evidence that recall involves elaboration—that the human mind transforms (rather than copies) past memories (Bartlett 1932). In addition, that which is out of awareness is not necessarily a seething cauldron of primitive instincts operating without logic. When a hypnotized subject allows "the unconscious" to talk, its voice, while perhaps novel and surprising, follows the usual rules of grammar and logic (cf. Lakoff, Chapter 4 in this volume). Similarly, although we control thoughts and feelings in various ways, it is unlikely that thought and emotion can be simply divorced. As indicated earlier, affect has a particular cognitive structure (Lakoff 1987; Piaget 1954/1981), and cognition invariably involves affect.

Can we come up with a better way to transform the folk metaphor of the mind? The distinction between implicit and explicit cognition (Kihlstrom 1987; Schachter 1987) and a consideration of the circumstances under which the two modes can be dissociated may be useful in this regard. Kihlstrom (1987) has elaborated the implicit/explicit distinction by separating cognition into several categories—memory, perception, thought, and learning. We will consider each of these briefly in turn (see also Cloitre, Chapter 3 in this volume).

## Implicit Versus Explicit Cognition

First, implicit memory has long been described in patients with neurological disorders who have amnesia (often involving lesions of the medial temporal lobe or diencephalon (Graf and Masson 1993; A. D. Milner and Rugg 1992; B. Milner et al. 1968; Roediger and Craik 1989; Shimamura 1989). For example, Korsakoff (1889) described an amnesic patient to whom he administered electric shocks during a session. Later, when Korsakoff returned carrying the shock apparatus, the patient accused him of coming to give him electric shocks. Similarly, Claparède (1911/1951) greeted an amnesic patient with a handshake, simultaneously pricking the patient with a pin. The patient later refused to shake the psychologist's hand, explaining that some people carry pins around with them. In these cases, despite the absence of an explicit memory of the traumatic event, there is clearly an implicit memory of the incident.

Subsequent empirical research on amnesic patients has confirmed a dissociation between explicit memory of a stimulus and implicit memory tasks (e.g., repetition priming or word-stem completion) (Warrington and Weiskrantz 1968). Dissociation of implicit and explicit memory is also found in nonimpaired subjects (Hintzman 1988; Richardson-Klavehn and Bjork 1988). Schachter (1987) and Reber (1993) have reviewed the variety of names used to designate these two kinds of memory—for example, procedural versus declarative (Anderson 1976; Cohen 1984), semantic versus episodic (Tulving 1972), working versus reference (Honig 1978), and cognitive versus semantic (Warrington and Weiskrantz 1982). The implicit versus explicit designation has, however, become increasingly used (Graf and Masson 1993).

The concept of unconscious processing of perception goes at least as far back as Helmholtz (1867/1962), who held that visual perception depended on "unconscious inferences." The philosopher Pierce and his colleague Jastrow (1884) noted that subjects were able to judge, with significantly more than chance accuracy, slight differences in the weight of two objects that consciously seemed equally heavy. Poetzl (1917/1960) noted that although subjects were unaware of tachistoscopically presented stimuli, these stimuli would later appear in their dreams and associations. The construct of perceptual defense (Dixon 1971, 1981; Erdelyi 1974, 1985; Eriksen and Pierce 1968; Holender 1986; Merikle 1982) guided a great deal of subsequent empirical research.

More recent work (Bornstein and Pittman 1992) has used a variety of paradigms to assess perception without awareness. For example, visual-masking paradigms involve the presentation first of a stimulus A (subliminally) and then of a stimulus B (supraliminally). Although the A-stimulus is not consciously detected, there is evidence of its being processed. In an early study by Eagle (1959), the A-stimulus was a drawing of a boy performing either a benevolent or a malevolent act, whereas the B-stimulus was a boy with a neutral expression. Despite subjects' lack of awareness of the A-stimulus, its content clearly influenced their perceptions and judgments of the boy. Marcel concluded that a conscious percept "is obtained by a constructive act of fitting a perceptual hypothesis to its sensory source" (1983, p. 245).

Implicit thought has been studied by Bowers (1987). Subjects were presented with word triads and asked to think of a word that the triads had in common. Whereas some of the triads were in fact soluble, others were not. Despite not being able to give the solution for the soluble triad, subjects were able to determine which of the triads were soluble and insoluble with considerable accuracy.

Implicit learning was first shown in a series of studies by Reber and colleagues (Reber 1967, 1993). For example, subjects were asked to memorize a series of nonsense syllables produced by a formal algorithm. Despite not having been explicitly taught this algorithm, patients were subsequently able to distinguish grammatical from ungrammatical patterns. This result is perhaps less astonishing when one considers the ease with which children learn languages without formal grammar tuition.

Several other lines of research have branched out from such work (Cantor and Kihlstrom 1987; Langer 1978; Lewicki 1986; Nisbett and Ross 1980; Uleman and Bargh 1989; Wegner and Vallacher 1977), demonstrating the importance of unconscious influences on social cognition. Such research strongly suggests that the phenomena of implicit cognition are not limited to the laboratory.

At the same time, the neurobiological bases of implicit and explicit cognition have been increasingly studied. Much research (Prigatano and Schachter 1991) has focused on various neurological disorders, including visual disorders (inability to explicitly visualize objects in the impaired visual fields) (Weiskrantz et al. 1974), prosopagnosia (inability to explicitly recognize previously encountered faces as familiar) (De Haan et al. 1987; Tranel and Damasio 1985), hemianesthesia (inability to explicitly respond to touch on one side) (Paillard et al. 1983), and hemineglect (inability to explicitly attend to stimuli in one visual field) (Volpe et al. 1979). In each of these instances, implicit recognition of stimuli has been demonstrated. Similarly, studies in patients with acquired dyslexia and aphasia demonstrate that despite deficits on explicit tasks, patients show evidence of intact implicit processing (Andrewsky and Seron 1975; Milberg and Blumstein 1981; Shallice and Saffran 1986). Research work has attempted to go beyond this kind of neuropsychological paradigm in an effort to detail the specific neuroanatomical and neurochemical bases of implicit and explicit cognition (Nissen et al. 1987; Schachter 1992; Schachter et al. 1988).

The question next arises of whether dissociation of implicit and explicit cognition is also present in altered states of consciousness and in functional disorders. There is in fact evidence for the presence of such dissociation in hypnosis (Kihlstrom 1980), sleep (Evans 1979), and anesthesia (Kihlstrom and Schachter 1990). Patients in such states may not be explicitly aware of stimuli, but they are able to demonstrate implicit knowledge. Similarly, several reports exist of similar phenomena in functional disorders (Kihlstrom 1987). These include a description of a patient with functional anesthesia and paralysis who nonetheless learns a finger-withdrawal response in the affected area, of a functionally blind patient who displays discriminative responses to visual stimuli, and similar cases. Analogous findings have been seen in patients with functional amnesia and other dissociative disorders. For example, whereas alters in patients with dissociative identity disorder have been found not to demonstrate shared explicit memory, they nonetheless show evidence of shared implicit memory (Nissen et al. 1989).

Why do dissociations between implicit and explicit cognition occur? Several answers have been suggested. One has to do with normal developmental learning. Explicit cognition takes place only in later years, after maturation of the brain and mind (Eagle 1987). Indeed, Reber (1993) argues that the implicit cognitive system is evolutionarily older than the explicit cognitive system. Dissociation may, however, also reflect characteristics of the stimuli, with weak (tachistoscopic) stimuli being processed implicitly but not explicitly. Characteristics of the individual are also important. Neurological damage or altered states of consciousness (cf. Breuer and Freud 1893–1895/1955) may, for example, result in dissociation. Furthermore, explicit cognition is to some extent state dependent. For example, stimuli learned during a particular mood state are likely to be more readily recalled on explicit testing when that state is induced (Bower 1981). At the heart of the dynamic unconscious, however, lies an emphasis on psychological pain. Indeed, Janet (1889) posited that trauma results in dissociation of implicit and explicit memories. Nevertheless, dissociation of implicit and explicit cognition can clearly occur in the absence of trauma. Indeed, the possibility also exists that dissociation can be willed. Subjects are able to report pushing thoughts or feelings out of awareness (Cloitre, Chapter 3 in this volume), and a similar phenomenon occurs in hypnotic suggestion. A final possibility is that dissociation of implicit and explicit cognition has to do with whether or not self-schemas are involved in the information processing (Eagle 1987; Kihlstrom 1987). In the words of Klein (1976), repression is "the refusal to acknowledge the *meaning* of a tendency" (p. 274).

# Schemas

The construct of schemas has been widely used in cognitive science, psychodynamic theory, and cognitive-behavioral theory (Singer and Salovey 1991; Stein 1992). Theorists typically assume that schemas are organizations of conceptually related elements that represent a prototypical abstraction of these elements; that schemas gradually develop from past experience; and that schemas guide the organization of new information (Thorndyke and Hayes-Roth 1979). These assumptions, taken together with work on the implicit/explicit distinction, yield the concept that schemas may operate implicitly but not necessarily with the subject's awareness.

Consider, for example, a person who is brought up in a family in which instability and abuse are the norm. Such a person may develop a "mistrust schema" according to which others are likely to hurt, manipulate, and take advantage of him or her (Stein and Young 1992; Young 1990). Such a schema is not a purely cognitive entity; rather, it is likely to incorporate affects such as fear, shame, and anger. Insofar as the schema develops early and is central to the person's view of him- or herself and others, it is also likely to be relatively resistant to change, with later experience being processed in such a way that the schema is maintained.

It is notable that a patient who enters therapy with a maladaptive mistrust schema is unlikely to offer this as the presenting complaint. Instead, the therapist must infer the existence of the schema from the patient's thoughts and feelings, often as they manifest in the therapeutic relationship. One might say that the schema is operating implicitly, with little explicit awareness. An important part of the therapeutic work is therefore to point out the existence of the schema, the factors that trigger its activation, and its maladaptive effects, so that the development of more adaptive schemas can be facilitated.

Although personality disorder patients are particularly likely to have maladaptive schemas, all of us have cognitive-affective structures that determine our view of self and other. Maladaptive schemas are likely to be relatively rigid and inflexible and to interfere with interpersonal relationships. In contrast, the operation of cognitive-affective structures outside of awareness in everyday relationships is likely to facilitate social interaction insofar as such operation allows rapid and accurate processing of interpersonal information.

A concept of the implicit operation of person schemas clearly differs from the Freudian notion of the unconscious. The unconscious is not so much a seething cauldron of irrationality as an understandable patterning of cognition and affect that has developed from the past and that structures current experience. Similarly, there is no particular energy cost to having a particular schema operate implicitly; rather, there are simply the disadvantages that accrue from the use of a maladaptive schema.

A concept of implicit operation of person schemas also differs from the cognitive psychological notion of repression as transformation of symbols. Schemas cannot be conceptualized in terms of abstract algorithms; rather, they are embodied—they are cognitive-affective structures that gradually develop from inborn neural schemas that are molded during and triggered by particular social interactions (Gilbert 1992; Piaget 1952). In terms used in an earlier chapter (Stein, Chapter 1 in this volume), schema theory incorporates both mechanism and meaning.

## Controls

The term *cognitive control*, although coined within the ego psychology tradition (Klein 1958, 1976; Klein and Schlesinger 1949), is now commonly employed by cognitivists (Ingram and Kendall 1986). This term is useful in considering the different strategies that are available for controlling schema activation and avoidance.

Let us go back to the case of the person with a mistrust schema. This person may report chronic feelings of suspicion when new relationships begin. One day, however, the patient (say, a woman) may walk into the therapist's office and say that on the previous night she met a man, felt sort of numb, and impulsively agreed to sleep with him. She now feels devastated and cannot make sense of what happened.

The cognitive therapist may interpret this behavior in terms of schema avoidance (Young 1990). Closer examination of the sequence of events may reveal, for example, that the patient had initially decided that she would allow herself to be open to a new way of seeing men. Alternatively, the patient may have blocked the feelings usually associated with her mistrust schema—an interpretation that is consistent with her report of feeling numb. Such cognitive-affective schema avoidance may have occurred automatically or volitionally.

Another commonly used exemplar of schema avoidance is the patient with posttraumatic stress disorder. Let us return to the victim of a rape, who now takes a new route home. Although this person does not explicitly articulate her reasoning, an implicit memory of the trauma would seem to be operating. Indeed, Gudjonsson (1979) demonstrated electrodermal responses to "forgotten" events in a rape victim. In such cases, there would seem to be avoidance of the traumatic schema, perhaps with dissociation of the rape memory from self-schemas.

Schema avoidance may be seen as analogous to prototypical motor patterns. The folk metaphor of repression emphasized that thoughts and feelings are "pushed down," whereas Freud described repression as an attempt at flight (Cloitre, Chapter 3 in this volume). In words consistent with the view taken here, Rosenblatt and Thickstun (1977) characterized defense mechanisms as symbolic actions that are elaborated from motor sequences. Nevertheless, schema control may result in quite complex effects—leading, for example, to shifts in state of mind, shifts in self–other schemas, or shifts in mental events (Horowitz, Chapter 8 in this volume; Horowitz et al. 1990).

Once again, it should be emphasized that schema controls are not necessarily pathological; on the contrary, regulation of the activation of schemas is a universal phenomenon. Each of us adopts a distinctive set of cognitive-affective strategies. Different subsets of the population (e.g., obsessive versus hysterical individuals, men versus women), however, may tend to adopt one or another kind of strategy (Tannen 1991). Such strategies result in various forms of attentional and response bias (Cloitre 1992).

Once again, this view of schema controls differs from the Freudian notion of the unconscious. The decision to activate or avoid a schema is less a matter of physical energetics than a control strategy that may itself become automatized. Schema activation is not simply a matter of copying memories from the unconscious, but may involve schema transformation. Affect and cognition are not simply divorcible; rather, schema controls involve the regulation of cognitive-affective structures. Similarly, patients with different personality disorders do not simply repress either ideas or affects;

rather, they differ in the nature of their maladaptive schemas and cognitive-affective strategies.

The concept of schema controls also differs from the cognitive psychological notion of the unconscious as purely procedural. Schema controls are not simply abstract transformations; rather, these controls involve specific kinds of cognitive-affective processing, which are associated with particular brain embodiments and correlations (Schwartz 1990; Stein 1996) and which take place in particular social contexts. Again, in the terms used in an earlier chapter (Stein, Chapter 1 in this volume), a theory of schema control must incorporate both mechanism and meaning.

## Clinical Implications

The view of schema maintenance and avoidance briefly outlined here has clear clinical implications (Young 1990). Psychotherapy of patients with personality disorders can be viewed in terms of person-schema evaluation and change. Patients can be directly asked about typical schema-driven behaviors (e.g., mistrusting significant others); however, given that schemas may not be explicitly recognized, comprehensive schema evaluation requires the ongoing collection of thoughts and feelings, including those involving the therapeutic relationship.

An additional important focus of psychotherapy is the exploration of schema controls. Having established the existence of a maladaptive schema, important next steps include an investigation of factors that trigger schema activation, as well as of signs and symptoms that point to schema avoidance. Schema avoidance can then be gently confronted, and alternative cognitive-affective strategies encouraged. Once again, the therapeutic relationship is an important tool in this work; for example, a relationship that is experienced as safe may provide the patient freedom to recall traumatic memories.

Insofar as schemas are not simply cognitive structures, techniques that involve affect arousal (e.g., role playing, imagery) may be particularly helpful in activating relevant schemas (Greenberg and Safran 1987). Therapists can then begin the difficult work of making maladaptive schemas and controls less ego-syntonic, encouraging the patient to develop new cognitive-affective structures and strategies. Such change requires behavioral practice, the therapeutic relationship once again often providing a useful first place to practice new ways of interpersonal relating. Because core person schemas may be highly resistant to change, psychotherapy of personality disorders may need to be a relatively long-term process. Single traumatic memories that do not involve core self-schemas may, however, allow for a briefer therapy.

## Conclusion

Freud described a number of real phenomena, including such entities as posttraumatic stress pathology, obsessive-compulsive personality disorder, and histrionic personality disorder. His theory developed the folk metaphor of MIND as CONTAINER in a sophisticated and productive way. Nevertheless, psychoanalytic theory also retained some of the erroneous assumptions of the folk metaphor.

Cognitive psychology opens up a new way looking at repression, replacing Freud's outdated metapsychology with current computational models. Nevertheless, some cognitivists have attempted to understand psychopathology in terms of formal algorithms of symbol transformation. In doing so, they have lost some of the richer, embodied notions of mind developed by psychoanalysis.

In this chapter, we have attempted to approach the phenomena described by Freud, going beyond his metapsychology but retaining a focus on embodied cognition. Advances in understanding dissociation of implicit and explicit cognition and cognitivist work on schema and control theory provide new constructs for reframing the folk metaphor of repression. This reframing seeks to enable a discussion of the mechanisms of the mind that also considers how such mechanisms operate within a meaningful context.

Should the term *repression* be dropped? We don't think it can be, because it points to a key folk metaphor of the mind, one that is based on real phenomena (cf. Goldman 1993). Nevertheless, we do think that the metaphor entailed by the term *repression* is erroneous in a number of ways, and that a more sophisticated reconstruction of these phenomena is needed.

Further empirical work on the operation of schemas and controls in psychopathology is needed (Horowitz 1991). Cognitive science methodologies can be combined to investigate the complex psychobiological underpinnings of these constructs (Shevrin 1990). Such work on the phenomena of repression will in turn be helpful in integrating the cognitive and dynamic unconscious.

# References

Anderson JR: Language, Memory, and Thought. Hillsdale, NJ, Lawrence Erlbaum, 1976

Andrewsky EL, Seron X: Implicit processing of grammatical rules in a classical case of agrammatism. Cortex 11:379–390, 1975

Bartlett FC: Remembering: A Study in Experimental and Social Psychology. Cambridge, UK, Cambridge University Press, 1932

Bornstein RF, Pittman TS (eds): Perception Without Awareness: Cognitive, Clinical, and Social Perspectives. New York, Guilford, 1992

Bower GH: Mood and memory. Am Psychol 36:129–148, 1981

Bowers KS: Revisioning the unconscious. Canadian Psychology 28:93–104, 1987

Breuer J, Freud S: On the psychical mechanism of hysterical phenomena: preliminary communication (1893), in The Standard Edition of the Complete Psychological Works of Sigmund Freud, Vol 2. Translated and edited by Strachey J. London, Hogarth Press, 1955, pp 1–18

Breuer J, Freud S: Studies on hysteria (1893–1895), in The Standard Edition of the Complete Psychological Works of Sigmund Freud, Vol 2. Translated and edited by Strachey J. London, Hogarth Press, 1955, pp 1–306

Byrne D, Barry J, Nelson D: The revised repression-sensitization scale and its relationship to measures of self-description. Psychol Rep 13:323–334, 1963

Cantor N, Kihlstrom JF: Personality and Social Intelligence. Englewood Cliffs, NJ, Prentice-Hall, 1987

Claparède E: Recognition and "me-ness" (1911), in Organization and Pathology of Thought. Edited by Rapaport D. New York, Columbia University Press, 1951, pp 58–75

Cloitre M: Avoidance of emotional processing: a cognitive science perspective, in Cognitive Science and Clinical Disorders. Edited by Stein DJ, Young JE. San Diego, CA, Academic Press, 1992, pp 19–44

Cohen NJ: Preserved learning capacity in amnesia: evidence for multiple memory systems, in Neuropsychology of Memory. Edited by Squire LR, Butters N. New York, Guilford, 1984, pp 83–102

Davis PJ, Schwartz GE: Repression and the inaccessibility of affective memories. J Pers Soc Psychol 52:155–162, 1987

De Haan EHF, Young AW, Newcombe F: Face recognition without awareness. Cognitive Neuropsychology 4:385–415, 1987

Dixon NF: Subliminal Processing: The Nature of a Controversy. New York, McGraw-Hill, 1971

Dixon NF: Preconscious Processing. New York, Wiley, 1981

Dollard J, Miller N: Personality and Psychotherapy. New York, McGraw-Hill, 1950

Eagle MN: The effects of subliminal stimuli of aggressive content upon conscious cognition. Journal of Personality 27:48–64, 1959

Eagle MN: The psychoanalytic and the cognitive unconscious, in Theories of the Unconscious and Theories of the Self. Edited by Stern R. Hillsdale, NJ, Lawrence Erlbaum, 1987, pp 155–190

Ellenberger HF: The Rediscovery of the Unconscious: The History and Evolution of Dynamic Psychiatry. New York, Basic Books, 1970

Erdelyi MH: A new look at the new look: perceptual defense and vigilance. Psychol Rev 81:1–25, 1974

Erdelyi MH: Psychoanalysis: Freud's Cognitive Psychology. New York, WH Freeman, 1985

Erdelyi MH: Repression, reconstruction, and defense: history and integration of the psychoanalytic and experimental frameworks, in Repression and Dissociation: Implications for Personality Theory, Psychopathology, and Health. Edited by Singer JL. Chicago, IL, University of Chicago Press, 1990, pp 1–32

Erdelyi MH, Goldberg B: Let's not sweep repression under the rug: toward a cognitive psychology of repression, in Functional Disorders of Memory. Edited by Kihlstrom JF, Evans FJ. Hillsdale, NJ, Lawrence Erlbaum, 1979, pp 355–402

Eriksen C, Pierce J: Defense mechanisms, in Handbook of Personality Theory and Research. Edited by Borgatta E, Lambert W. Chicago, IL, Rand McNally, 1968

Evans FJ: Hypnosis and sleep: techniques for exploring cognitive activity during sleep, in Hypnosis: Developments in Research and New Perspectives. Edited by Fromm E, Shorr RE. New York, Aldine, 1979, pp 139–184

Faught WS, Colby KM, Parkinson RC: Inferences, affects, and intentions in a model of paranoia. Cognitive Psychology 9:153–187, 1977

Freud S: A case of successful treatment by hypnotism: with some remarks on the origin of hysterical symptoms through "counter-will" (1892–1893), in The Standard Edition of the Complete Psychological Works of Sigmund Freud, Vol 1. Translated and edited by Strachey J. London, Hogarth Press, 1966, pp 115–128

Freud S: The neuro-psychoses of defense (1894), in The Standard Edition of the Complete Psychological Works of Sigmund Freud, Vol 3. Translated and edited by Strachey J. London, Hogarth Press, 1962, pp 41–68

Freud S: On the history of the psychoanalytic movement (1915), in The Standard Edition of the Complete Psychological Works of Sigmund Freud, Vol 14. Translated and edited by Strachey J. London, Hogarth Press, 1957, pp 7–66

Freud S: Repression (1915), in The Standard Edition of the Complete Psychological Works of Sigmund Freud, Vol 14. Translated and edited by Strachey J. London, Hogarth Press, 1957, pp 141–158

Freud S: Inhibitions, symptoms, and anxiety (1926), in The Standard Edition of the Complete Psychological Works of Sigmund Freud, Vol 20. Translated and edited by Strachey J. London, Hogarth Press, 1959, pp 75–175

Gilbert P: Human Nature and Suffering. New York, Guilford, 1992

Goldman A: Consciousness, folk psychology, and cognitive science. Consciousness and Cognition 2:364–382, 1993

Graf P, Masson MEJ (eds): Implicit Memory: New Directions in Cognition, Development and Neuropsychology. Hillsdale, NJ, Lawrence Erlbaum, 1993

Greenberg LS, Safran J: Emotion in Psychotherapy. New York, Guilford, 1987

Gudjonsson GH: The use of electrodermal responses in a case of amnesia. Med Sci Law 19:138–140, 1979

Hammond CD (ed): Hypnotic Induction and Suggestion: An Introductory Manual. Des Plaines, IL, American Society of Clinical Hypnosis, 1992

Helmholtz H: Treatise on Physiological Optics, Vol 3 (1867). New York, Dover, 1962

Hintzman DL: Human learning and memory: connections and dissociations. Annu Rev Psychol 41:109–139, 1988

Holender D: Semantic activation without conscious identification in dichotic listening, parafoveal vision, and visual masking: a survey and appraisal. Behavioral and Brain Sciences 9:1–66, 1986

Holmes DS: The evidence for repression: an examination of sixty years of research, in Repression and Dissociation: Implications for Personality Theory, Psychopathology, and Health. Edited by Singer JL. Chicago, IL, University of Chicago Press, 1990, pp 85–102

Honig WK: Studies of working memory in the pigeon, in Cognitive Processes in Animal Behavior. Edited by Hulse SH, Fowler H, Honig WK. Hillsdale, NJ, Lawrence Erlbaum, 1978, pp 211–248

Horowitz MJ (ed): Person Schemas and Maladaptive Interpersonal Patterns. Chicago, IL, University of Chicago Press, 1991

Horowitz MJ, Markman HC, Stinson CH, et al: A classification theory of defense, in Repression and Dissociation: Implications for Personality Theory, Psychopathology, and Health. Edited by Singer JL. Chicago, IL, University of Chicago Press, 1990, pp 61–84

Ingram RE, Kendall PC: Cognitive clinical psychology: implications of an information-processing perspective, in Information Processing Approaches to Clinical Psychology. New York, Academic Press, 1986, pp 261–284

Janet P: Psychological Automatisms. Paris, Alcan, 1889

Jung CJ: Studies in Word Association. London, Heinemann, 1918 (originally published in 1906)

Kihlstrom JF: Posthypnotic amnesia for recently learned material: Interactions with "episodic" and "semantic" memory. Cognitive Psychology 12:227–251, 1980

Kihlstrom JF: The cognitive unconscious. Science 237:1445–1452, 1987

Kihlstrom JF, Schachter DL: Anaesthesia, amnesia, and the cognitive unconscious, in Memory and Awareness during Anaesthesia. Edited by Bonke B, Fitch W, Millar K. Amsterdam, Netherlands, Swets & Zeitlinger, 1990, pp 22–44

Klein GS: Cognitive control and motivation, in Assessment of Human Motives. New York, Holt, Rinehart & Winston, 1958

Klein GS: Psychoanalytic Theory: An Exploration of Essentials. New York, International Universities Press, 1976

Klein GS, Schlesinger HJ: Where is the perceiver in perceptual theory? Journal of Personality 18:32–47, 1949

Korsakoff SS: Etude medico-psychologique sur une forme des maladies de la memoire. Revue Philosophique 28:501–530, 1889

Lakoff G: Women, Fire, and Dangerous Things: What Categories Reveal About the Mind. Chicago, IL, University of Chicago Press, 1987

Langer E: Rethinking the role of thought in social interaction, in New Directions in Attribution Theory, Vol 2. Edited by Harvey J, Ickes W, Kidd R. Hillsdale, NJ, Lawrence Erlbaum, 1978

Lewicki P: Nonconscious Social Information Processing. New York, Academic Press, 1986

MacKinnon D, Dukes W: Repression in Psychology in the Making. Edited by Postman L. New York, Knopf, 1964

Marcel AJ: Conscious and unconscious perception: an approach to the relations between phenomenal experience and perceptual processes. Cognitive Psychology 15:238–300, 1983

McClelland JL, Rumelhart DE, PDP Research Group (eds): Parallel Distributed Processing: Explorations in the Microstructure of Cognition, Vol 2: Psychological and Biological Models. Cambridge, MA, MIT Press, 1986

Merikle PM: Unconscious perception revisited. Perception and Psychophysics 31:298–301, 1982

Milberg W, Blumstein SE: Lexical decision and aphasia: evidence for semantic processing. Brain Lang 14:371–385, 1981

Milner AD, Rugg MD (eds): The Neuropsychology of Consciousness. New York, Academic Press, 1992

Milner B, Corkin S, Teuber HL: Further analysis of the hippocampal amnesic syndrome: 14-year follow-up study of H.M. Neuropsychologica 6:215–234, 1968

Nisbett RE, Ross L: Human Inference: Strategies and Shortcomings of Social Judgment. Englewood Cliffs, NJ, Prentice-Hall, 1980

Nissen MJ, Knopman DS, Schachter DL: Neurochemical dissociation of memory systems. Neurology 37:789–794, 1987

Nissen MJ, Ross JL, Willingham DB, et al: Memory and awareness in a patient with multiple personality disorder. Brain Cogn 8:117–134, 1989

Norman DA: Cognition in the head and in the world: an introduction to the special issue on situated action. Cognition 17:1–6, 1993

Paillard J, Michel F, Stelmach G: Localization without content: a tactile analogue of "blind sight." Arch Neurology 40:548–551, 1983

Piaget J: The Origins of Intelligence in Children. New York, International Universities Press, 1952

Piaget J: Intelligence and Affectivity: Their Relationship During Child Development (1954). Palo Alto, CA, Annual Reviews, 1981

Pierce CS, Jastrow J: On small differences in sensation. Memoirs of the National Academy of Science 3:75–83, 1884

Poetzl O: The relationships between experimentally induced dream images and indirect vision (1917), in Preconscious Stimulation in Dreams, Associations, and Images: Classical Studies (Psychological Issues 2, monograph 7). Edited by Fisher C. New York, International Universities Press, 1960, pp 46–106

Prigatano GP, Schachter DL (eds): Awareness of Deficit After Brain Injury: Clinical and Theoretical Issues. New York, Oxford University Press, 1991

Rapaport D: Emotions and Memory. New York, International Universities Press, 1942

Reber AS: Implicit learning of artificial grammars. Journal of Verbal Learning and Verbal Behavior 77:317–327, 1967

Reber AS: Implicit Learning and Tacit Knowledge: An Essay on the Cognitive Unconscious. New York, Oxford University Press, 1993

Richardson-Klavehn A, Bjork RA: Measures of memory. Annu Rev Psychol 39:475–543, 1988

Roediger HL, Craik FIM (eds): Varieties of Memory and Consciousness: Essays in Honour of Endel Tulving. Hillsdale, NJ, Lawrence Erlbaum, 1989

Rosenblatt AD, Thickstun JT: Energy, information, and motivation: a revision of psychoanalytic theory. J Am Psychoanal Assoc 25:529–558, 1977

Rumelhart DE, McClelland JL, PDP Research Group (eds): Parallel Distributed Processing: Explorations in the Microstructure of Cognition, Vol 1: Foundations. Cambridge, MA, MIT Press, 1986

Schachter DL: Implicit memory: history and current status. J Exp Psychol Learn Mem Cogn 13:501–518, 1987

Schachter DL: Understanding implicit memory: a cognitive neuroscience approach. Am Psychol 47:559–569, 1992

Schachter DL, McAndrews MP, Moscovitch M: Access to consciousness: dissociations between implicit and explicit knowledge in neuropsychological syndromes, in Thought without Language. Edited by Weiskrantz L, London, Oxford University Press, 1988, pp 242–278

Schwartz G: Psychobiology of repression and health: a systems approach, in Repression and Dissociation: Implications for Personality Theory, Psychopathology, and Health. Edited by Singer JL. Chicago, IL, University of Chicago Press, 1990, pp 405–434

Shallice T, Saffran E: Lexical processing in the absence of explicit word identification: evidence from a letter-by-letter reader. Cognitive Neuropsychology 3:429–458, 1986

Shevrin H: Subliminal perception and repression, in Repression and Dissociation: Implications for Personality Theory, Psychopathology, and Health. Edited by Singer JL. Chicago, IL, University of Chicago Press, 1990, pp 471–496

Shimamura AP: Disorders of memory: the cognitive science perspective, in Handbook of Neuropsychology. Edited by Boller F, Grafman J. Amsterdam, Netherlands, Elsevier, 1989, pp 35–73

Simon H: Motivational and emotional controls of cognition. Psychol Rev 74:29–39, 1967

Singer JL (ed): Repression and Dissociation: Implications for Personality Theory, Psychopathology, and Health. Chicago, IL, University of Chicago Press, 1990

Singer JL, Salovey P: Organized knowledge structures and personality: person schemas, self schemas, prototypes, and scripts, in Person Schemas and Maladaptive Interpersonal Patterns. Edited by Horowitz MJ. Chicago, IL, University of Chicago Press, 1991, pp 33–79

Singer JL, Sincoff JB: Beyond repression and the defenses, in Repression and Dissociation: Implications for Personality Theory, Psychopathology, and Health. Edited by Singer JL. Chicago, IL, University of Chicago Press, 1990, pp 471–496

Sloman A: Motives, mechanisms, and emotions. Cognition and Emotion 1:217–233, 1987

Stein DJ: Schemas in the cognitive and clinical sciences: an integrative construct. Journal of Psychotherapy Integration 2:45–63, 1992

Stein DJ: Cognitive science models of impulsivity and compulsivity, in Impulsivity and Compulsivity. Edited by Oldham J, Hollander E, Skodol AE. Washington, DC, American Psychiatric Press, 1996, pp 97–118

Stein DJ: Implications of the complexity of psychoanalysis for cognitive science, in Cognition and Psychodynamics: New Perspectives. Edited by Kurtzman H. New York, Oxford University Press (in press)

Stein DJ, Young JE: A schema-focused approach to personality disorders, in Cognitive Science and Clinical Disorders. Edited by Stein DJ, Young JE. San Diego, CA, Academic Press, 1992, pp 272–289

Suppes P, Warren H: On the generation and classification of defence mechanisms. Int J Psychoanal 56:405–414, 1975

Swanson DR: A critique of psychic energy as an explanatory concept. J Am Psychoanal Assoc 25:603–633, 1977

Tannen D: You Just Don't Understand: Women and Men in Conversation. New York, Ballantine Books, 1991

Thorndyke PW, Hayes-Roth B: The use of schemata in the acquisition and transference of knowledge. Cognitive Psychology 11:82–106, 1979

Tranel D, Damasio AR: Knowledge without awareness: an autonomic index of facial recognition by prosopagnosics. Science 228:1453–1454, 1985

Tulving E: Episodic and semantic memory, in Organization of Memory. Edited by Tulving E, Donaldson W. New York, Academic Press, 1972, pp 381–403

Uleman JS, Bargh JA (eds): Unintended Thought. New York, Guilford, 1989

Volpe BT, Ledoux JE, Gazzaniga MS: Information processing of visual stimuli in an "extinguished" field. Nature 282:722–724, 1979

Warrington EK, Weiskrantz L: New method of testing long-term retention with special reference to amnesic patients. Nature 217:972–974, 1968

Warrington EK, Weiskrantz L: Amnesia: a disconnection syndrome? Neuropsychologia 20:233–248, 1982

Wegman C: Psychoanalysis and Cognitive Psychology: A Formalization of Freud's Earliest Theory. London, Academic Press, 1985

Wegner DM, Vallacher RR: Implicit Psychology: An Introduction to Social Cognition. New York, Oxford University Press, 1977

Weiskrantz L, Warrington EK, Sanders MD, et al: Visual capacity in the hemianopic field following a restricted occipital ablation. Brain 97:709–728, 1974

Wollheim R: The Mind and Its Depths. Cambridge, MA, Harvard University Press, 1993

Young JE: Cognitive Therapy for Personality Disorders: A Schema-Focused Approach. Sarasota, FL, Professional Resource Exchange, 1990

Zeigarnik B: Das Behalten non erledigten und unerledigten Handlungen. Psychologie Forschung 9:1–85, 1927

# Chapter 7

# *Dissociated Cognition and Disintegrated Experience*

David Spiegel, M.D., and David Li, M.D.

---

At first blush, dissociation seems to be a strange phenomenon, defying common sense. Memories that should be available are lost, identity is fragmented, consciousness is altered. At times, the phenomena are so vivid that they seem more the product of acting than actual mental states, and at other times, they are so well hidden that neither patient nor family or friends know that they are occurring. Yet dissociative phenomena are ubiquitous in time and place. They have been reported for centuries and are observed throughout the world. These disaggregations of mental function are often seen in association with trauma. Elements of identity, memory, perception, and consciousness are segregated one from another, divided in function—but not of necessity, since their segregation is potentially reversible through techniques such as hypnosis. This aspect leads some to assume that such phenomena are feigned or induced by suggestion rather than real. Yet what makes dissociative phenomena so interesting is that they are at the boundary of consciousness, often functioning independently of and yet capable of being brought under conscious control.

## Dissociation in Memory

The distinctions between explicit and implicit memory put forward in this volume are illustrative. Experimental instructions to suppress recollection will reduce explicit but not implicit recall.

Schachter (1992) has observed that the alters in a patient with dissociative identity disorder will have obvious deficits in explicit memory but will have a common pool of implicit recollection. Although implicit memory is by nature relatively less "conscious" than explicit memory, explicit episodes clearly lead to the creation of implicit memory stores. Furthermore, the automaticity typical of implicit memory recall can be produced in hypnotic states in which instructed motor activity comes to seem instinctive rather than volitional (D. Spiegel et al. 1993; H. Spiegel and D. Spiegel 1978/1987).

Indeed, the phenomenon of early-childhood amnesia demonstrates the plausibility of the notion that information can be available but not accessible. Most of the learning that occurs during the first 4 years of life turns out to be implicit rather than explicit. We acquire a number of skills, ranging from language and motor skills to developing a coherent perceptual-organizational structure and schemas for object relations, yet we have little in the way of an explicit recollection of these events. While the occurrence of early-childhood amnesia is often used to attack the credibility of any recovered memories, the phenomenon also serves to illustrate that a variety of experiences may influence people without their having conscious recollection of them.

## Dissociation and Connectionism

Dissociation seems to be a strange or marginal phenomenon, and it can be understood not so much as an aberration but as a logical outcome of information-processing systems that are built bottom-up rather than top-down. Connectionism (i.e., parallel distributed processing [PDP] theory) holds first of all that memories are created—and perceptions processed—on the basis of patterns of co-occurrence of activation in neural networks (McClelland et al. 1986; Rumelhart et al. 1986) rather than through a top-down symbolic processor that neatly files percepts, memories, and cognitions in the appropriate categories. The second premise of PDP theory is that multiple information-processing events occur in parallel. This conceptualization makes integration of information problematic rather than routine. When multiple independent subsystems operate simultaneously, the relationships among them become problematic. One way of attempting to resolve this problem is Baars' (1988) *global workspace model*, in which various subunits compete for access to the serial processor, which can broadcast throughout the system, something like the sound-amplified rostrum in a legislative chamber. Rules for access to this general broadcasting system can allow for the orderly sharing of information, but situations may occur in which the units continue to compete rather than cooperate, in which one schema is diametrically opposed to another, or in which the affective connotation of a given schema profoundly and adversely influences the affective associations of other schemas. In such situations, time sharing may not progress smoothly, and competition among the units leads to an inability to broadcast information generally throughout the system.

## Trauma and Dissociation

Trauma is often the setting in which such a breakdown occurs. The experience of being made to feel helpless and degraded—for example, in victimization from sexual assault or natural disaster—causes intense negative affect and conflicts with a sense of the self as being in control and worthwhile. Some individuals can work through and reconcile these differences, seeing the experience as a terrible piece of history but not as determining their overall self-schema. Others desperately cling to the fantasy of being in control, often at the price of excessive and inappropriate guilt over imagined responsibility for events that were in fact uncontrollable. The helpless self is warded off and fundamentally incompatible with the invulnerable one. In such situations, integration of the conflicting elements is not achieved, and dissociation results in a failure to reconcile conflicting subunits.

These conflicting roles can be seen in the self-schemas of children subjected to sexual or physical abuse by parents. Such children are placed into dual roles that cannot easily be reconciled: dependent children who need and want love from their parents and victims of the parents' sadistic self-absorption, wishing to be good but treated as being bad, wishing to be comforted but receiving periodic pain and humiliation. Some resolve this dilemma by becoming these incompatible opposites: children who are ingratiatingly good but who feel evil and deserving of punishment, victims yet persons so powerful that they can choose—and, indeed, *arrange*—their victimhood. In this sense, such children experience a true double bind, as described by Bateson (1972; D. Spiegel 1986). A double bind involves a primary injunction suggesting one thing, a secondary injunction suggesting the opposite, and a prohibition on discussing the inconsistency. A child must be good but is treated as if she were bad, must be in total control of her emotions at all times but is rendered helpless. The failure to reconcile the differences tends to exaggerate them over time, so that the personality, identities, or mental states of a patient with dissociative identity disorder become caricatures—one pathetic and helpless, another hostile and uncaring. The problem is not having more than one personality; rather, it is having less than one personality.

There is growing evidence that dissociation occurs, especially in the aftermath of trauma. Recent research has found high frequencies of dissociative symptoms—such as numbing, amnesia, depersonalization, and derealization—in the wake of earthquakes (Cardeña and Spiegel 1993) and firestorms (Koopman et al. 1994), in those who have witnessed an execution (Freinkel et al. 1994), and in Vietnam theater veterans (Marmar et al. 1994). Whereas the traditional focus in the study of the aftermath of trauma has involved anxiety symptoms, this recent work suggests that dissociative and anxiety symptoms co-occur—and that, indeed, the presence of dissociative symptoms places individuals at risk for the later development of posttraumatic stress disorder (PTSD). DSM-IV (American Psychiatric Association 1994) contains a new diagnostic category, "acute stress disorder," which involves symptoms of numbing, depersonalization, derealization, amnesia, and stupor, along with intrusive memories, avoidance, and hyperarousal. Early detection of such symptoms may be helpful in preventing later PTSD (Koopman et al. 1994). Trauma represents an extreme discontinuity in experience that may indeed be reflected in discontinuities in mental function, a disaggregation of self-schemas and mental states that corresponds to the sudden disconnection imposed by the traumatic event itself. Traumatic experience forces the individual from one mood state to another, from a state of control over the body to helplessness, and this stress may later be repeated—once control over the body has been regained—in a loss of control over the mind. Indeed, dissociative symptoms may initially protect against an overwhelming sense of helplessness and loss of control. By detaching oneself from the pain and helplessness, an initial sense of control is maintained. Many rape victims report floating above their bodies, feeling sorry for the person being assaulted beneath them. This is an archetypal dissociative experience that may initially have an adaptive purpose in protecting the person from being overwhelmed by the reality of the traumatic event as it is occurring. However, the very success of such a defense may result in its exclusive use in preference to the difficult but necessary grief work of integrating competing and often irreconcilable schemas and memories (Lindemann 1944).

A review of the literature on reactions to trauma reveals that such experiences of mental detachment are not uncommon. Prison guards being beaten during a prison riot felt no pain (Noyes and Slyman 1978–1979). Numbness descended on victims of the North Sea oil disaster (Holen 1993). Depersonalization and derealization was reportedly common among victims of the Ash Wednesday Bush Fires (A. C. McFarlane 1986; S. McFarlane 1988). Solomon and Mikulincer (1988) found that numbing in the immediate aftermath of combat was the single best predictor of later PTSD among Israeli soldiers. The intrusive memories, avoidance, and hyperarousal characteristic of PTSD are also consistent with this connectionist point of view: the competition among unreconciled mental states; the intrusion of the traumatic memory, causing disequilibrium; and the loss of pleasure in usually pleasurable activities, as an implicit consequence of the traumatic experience.

# A Connectionist Model of Traumatic Dissociation

We have attempted to model this dissociative reaction to trauma in PDP terms (Li and Spiegel 1992) using a backpropagation model. In this model, traumatic input is symbolized by multiple inputs from one unit. Such input tends to make it difficult for the network to solve the problem of reaching a global minimum by balancing competing input unit relationships. Rather, such "traumatized" networks frequently become stuck in a local minimum as a result of being unable to distribute attention relatively equally across all of the input units, in essence paying more attention to some than to others. We have attempted to provide "therapy" for such networks by redirecting the networks' attention to these traumatic inputs and thus helping them to redistribute attention more broadly. In some cases, the networks were then able to achieve a global minimum. Intense and uneven input seems capable of traumatizing these networks, making it difficult for them to carry out their usual function of balancing input and reflecting the total pattern of activation rather than only certain portions of it. Rumelhart, McClelland, and colleagues (1986) have noted that traumatic amnesia could easily be modeled in PDP terms. A single input can cause disequilibrium in the network even though the overall pattern of activation may remain relatively unchanged. The memory is potentially available but not accessible. The basic pattern of activation is present, but the network has not solved its overall problem or reached a global minimum. Implicit activation could occur in the absence of explicit recollection. In this model, dissociative amnesia would be explained as follows: Memory traces for traumatic events exist, but either they are not identified with self (Kihlstrom 1987; Kihlstrom and Hoyt 1990) or self cannot emerge as the mediating factor across this variety of patterns (D. Spiegel 1990).

From this point of view, the notion of self is an emergent property defined by the network of relationships maintained. If the domain of networks being integrated is smaller or fragmented, the definition of self may be influenced such that, in a patient with dissociative identity disorder, certain types of experience, emotion, or relationships become inconsistent with a given set of memories or self-schemas. The passive personality cannot integrate information about assertiveness and interpersonal control. The hostile personality finds empathy and caring about others ridiculous and dangerous. Thus, the domain of memories, experiences, and intentions is restricted, and identity becomes fragmented. Just as the identity of a congressperson is defined, in part, by his or her constituency, to borrow terminology from Baars' global workspace model, so the type of consciousness and self-identity that emerges in the global workspace is defined by the domains of the competing input units that are represented.

Trauma is very difficult to integrate into awareness and seems to exacerbate an inherent problem in a connectionist system: overall integration. However, as illustrated by a number of other chapters in this book, clinical realities, even in extreme situations, may be explained in terms quite compatible with modern cognitive theory. Unconscious mental processing is not a speculative phenomenon; rather, it is a necessity for an extraordinarily complex system that manages enormous amounts of information. In order to remember, we cannot possibly remember how we remember. This means that automaticity (i.e., independence of subsystems not only allows us to remember, perceive, analyze, and identify ourselves but also provides opportunities for less-than-optimal or smooth functioning of these processes. Dissociation is the exception that proves the rule of connectionism.

A fundamental contribution of connectionist models is that they allow us to account for the approximate nature of human learning as distinct from the miss-is-as-good-as-a-mile nature of simple computer computation. Computer efforts at image recognition, for example, have been limited by this difficulty (humans, by contrast, are highly proficient in pattern recognition), and PDP network models have been helpful in addressing this problem. This bottom-up construction of pattern recognition means that the identification of a given image is a product of a series of associations rather than the result of a predetermined category. This means that in such a model, self-identity would not automatically be incorporated into an experience but rather might emerge only as other units consistent with the reinforcement of self-identity were activated. This could be true not only of traumatic input but also of any discontinuity in experience—for example, role changes such as graduating from school, getting married, taking on a new job, or becoming a parent. Because they are at variance with earlier aspects of identity, all of these changes involve the encoding of experiences that are "not me." Over time, the new experiences become more selflike and are linked more with previous aspects of self-identity. Dissociation of mental contents, and especially of identity or memory, is therefore consistent with a connectionist model that requires constant reconstruction of the context of memory through patterns of reactivation of input units. If, as is now known, memory is constitutive rather than restorative, the identification of self with memory is one of the components that needs to be continually reconstructed. It is therefore possible that situations could occur in which a person stored a memory as though it had happened not to him- or herself but rather to someone else, so that a request for personal history could activate a chain of networks that might not include the event in question. If the organizational logic of PDP networks consists simply of patterns of co-occurrence, then self-identity may or may not co-occur in any given instance. In addition, retrieval processes are very much influenced by the pattern of associations. Retrieval can be affected by external factors such as suggestion (D. Spiegel 1995) or by internal processes that make access to certain kinds of information dependent on specific associations. In essence, memories stored as patterns of activation that are missing certain elements, such as self-identification or affect, may lack the kinds of "hooks" that would respond to a search strategy. Experiencing oneself as numb or empty during an assault, for example, might leave the affect-related components of the experience/memory stored separately. Activating the memory might require a search for expected affect that is not connected with the content, thereby frustrating the search. On the other hand, the terror may be activated, thereby threatening current homeostasis.

# Conclusion

Distortions in memory, identity, and consciousness, as seen in the dissociative disorders, can be viewed as inevitable consequences of a system that must continually reinvent itself, reestablishing the connections between identity and memory, and very much influenced by any distortions in consciousness that occur as memories are encoded, stored, or retrieved. In this sense, identity is constantly reconstructed rather than assumed, and disturbances of it are expectable. Similarly, these models make clear how implicit information can have an effect even though there is no conscious awareness of it. The pattern of activations may occur without being linked to a conscious memory identified with self, which is indeed the way most implicit memories seem to work. The content of memories is activated and used even though the explicit episodes that led to the memories' encoding are not available. Thus, connectionist models can account not only for perceptual and memory processing but also for specific failures in this processing associated with traumatic experience.

# References

American Psychiatric Association: Diagnostic and Statistical Manual of Mental Disorders, 4th Edition. Washington, DC, American Psychiatric Association, 1994

Baars BJ: A Cognitive Theory of Consciousness. New York, Cambridge University Press, 1988

Bateson G: Steps to an Ecology of Mind. New York, Ballantine, 1972

Cardeña E, Spiegel D: Dissociative reactions to the Bay Area earthquake. Am J Psychiatry 150:474–478, 1993

Freinkel A, Koopman C, Spiegel D: Dissociative symptoms in media eyewitnesses of execution. Am J Psychiatry 151:1335–1339, 1994

Holen A: The North Sea oil rig disaster, in International Handbook of Traumatic Stress Syndromes. Edited by Wilson JP, Raphael B. New York, Plenum, 1993, pp 471–478

Kihlstrom JF: The cognitive unconscious. Science 237:1445–1452, 1987

Kihlstrom JF, Hoyt IP: Repression, dissociation and hypnosis, in Repression and Dissociation: Implications for Personality Theory, Psychopathology, and Health. Edited by Singer JL. Chicago, IL, University of Chicago Press, 1990, pp 181–208

Koopman C, Classen C, Spiegel D: Predictors of posttraumatic stress symptoms among Oakland/Berkeley firestorm survivors. Am J Psychiatry 151:888–894, 1994

Li D, Spiegel D: A neural network model of dissociative disorders. Psychiatric Annals 22:144–147, 1992

Lindemann E: Symptomatology and management of acute grief. Am J Psychiatry 101:141–148, 1944

Marmar CR, Weiss DS, Schlenger WE, et al: Peritraumatic dissociation and posttraumatic stress in male Vietnam theater veterans. Am J Psychiatry 151:902–907, 1994

McClelland JL, Rumelhart DE, PDP Research Group (eds): Parallel Distributed Processing: Explorations in the Microstructure of Cognition, Vol 2: Psychological and Biological Models. Cambridge, MA, MIT Press, 1986

McFarlane AC: Posttraumatic morbidity of a disaster: a study of cases presenting for psychiatric treatment. J Nerv Ment Dis 174:4–13, 1986

McFarlane S: The longitudinal course of posttraumatic morbidity: the range of outcomes and their predictors. J Nerv Ment Dis 176:30–39, 1988

Noyes R, Slyman DJ: The subjective response to life-threatening danger. Omega 9:313–321, 1978–1979

Rumelhart DE, McClelland JL, PDP Research Group (eds): Parallel Distributed Processing: Explorations in the Microstructure of Cognition, Vol 1: Foundations. Cambridge, MA, MIT Press, 1986

Schachter D: Understanding implicit memory: a cognitive neuroscience approach. Am Psychol 47:559–569, 1992

Soloman Z, Mikulincer M: Psychological sequelae of war: a two-year follow-up study of Israeli combat stress reaction (CSR) casualties. J Nerv Ment Dis 176:264–269, 1988

Spiegel D: Dissociation, double binds, and post-traumatic stress in multiple personality disorder, in Treatment of Multiple Personality Disorder. Edited by Braun B. Washington, DC, American Psychiatric Press, 1986, pp 63–77

Spiegel D: Hypnosis, dissociation, and trauma: hidden and overt observers, in Repression and Dissociation: Implications for Personality Theory, Psychopathology, and Health. Edited by Singer JL. Chicago, IL, University of Chicago Press, 1990, pp 121–142

Spiegel D: Hypnosis and suggestion, in Memory Distortion: How Minds, Brains, and Societies Reconstruct the Past. Edited by Schachter DL, Coyle JT, Fischbach GD, et al. Cambridge, MA, Harvard University Press, 1995, pp 129–149

Spiegel D, Frischolz EJ, Spira J: Functional disorders of memory, in American Psychiatric Press Review of Psychiatry, Vol 12. Edited by Oldham JM, Riba MB, Tasman A. Washington, DC, American Psychiatric Press, 1993, pp 747–782

Spiegel H, Spiegel D: Trance and Treatment: Clinical Uses of Hypnosis. New York, Basic Books, 1978 (reprinted by American Psychiatric Press, Washington, DC, 1987)

# Chapter 8

# Cognitive Psychodynamics: The Clinical Use of States, Person Schemas, and Defensive Control Process Theories

Mardi J. Horowitz, M.D.

P sychoanalysis provides a window to unconscious aspects of the mind. Such windows help us to understand the "whys" behind symptom formation. In turn, cognitive science provides a way of explaining how information from the immediate world combines with internal knowledge structures to alter both the world and the mind. Modern psychiatry combines both perspectives, arriving at a cognitive-psychodynamic synthesis for its psychological domain and integrating that domain with its biological, sociological, and anthropological domains.

Clinicians can use such integrations in case formulation. Dysfunctional beliefs and impaired information-processing styles can be identified and specific treatment plans made. The result can be effective attention-focusing techniques in psychotherapy. A configurational analysis system of formulation, to be presented in this chapter, is an example of such integration. This system uses states, person schemas, and defensive control processes as organizing principles.

## Rationale for Case Formulation

Our diagnostic system, DSM-IV (American Psychiatric Association 1994), is a descriptive one; it does not usefully guide clinicians toward a plan of *how* to alter the causes of symptoms. A static system of symptom menus such as DSM-IV must be supplemented with case formulation in order to plan individual treatments.

A system is needed that can provide a picture of repetitive maladaptive behavioral patterns and internal irrational meanings. The goal of treatment, then, is to modify both behaviors and dysfunctional beliefs.

One obstacle to lucid case formulation is the complexity and state-variability of symptoms and character traits. This obstacle can be surmounted by taking an approach that recognizes multiple states and cycles of states within each patient. Theoretical constructs of multiple selves and schemas of defense can help us arrive at an understanding of the reasons both for the existence of states and for recurrences of cyclical shifts in state. We can then clarify contradictions in belief, deficits in knowledge, and dilemmas of wish and fear.

State cycles can begin with positive emotion, as desired goals and good self- or relationship attributes are emphasized, and then shift to moods with negative emotions, as feared consequences and bad self- or other-person characteristics are emphasized. Some states in a cycle are defensive compromises that dull the edge of both wish and fear. Contradictions in beliefs of different states are not noises that obscure formulation of each patient's unitary theme; rather, they are the relevant "stuff" of discordancies in personality.

Applying cognitive science principles to the examination of unconscious information processing provides us with 1) a way to describe how shifts in state may occur; 2) a sketch of how preconscious processing of conflictual, stressful themes may be performed differently in separate parallel channels; and 3) a clear language to describe how preconscious information processing may affect conscious representation and physical action.

To recapitulate, we need to assume state variability in symptoms and character traits. Such a "states of mind" approach helps clinicians because it allows inference about how an individual's symptoms, defensive regulation, and sense of identity vary in different phases of a maladaptive cycle.

## Caveats Regarding Case Formulation

Any formulation should be regarded as open ended and as having areas of ambiguity and insecurity of evidence. One can allow for deep motives but not be able to accurately classify them. Similarly, childhood developmental lines tracing how dysfunctional identities and beliefs formed may remain obscure due to lack of information. The links and co-determinations among mind, brain, body, and society may be important but unclear. In many cases, one may be able to focus on psychological part-causations only at the here-and-now level, as is illustrated in the case example provided below.

## Formulation of an Illustrative Case

The four steps of configurational formulation are summarized in Table 8–1. Each of these will be discussed in turn, and a summary of the empirical evidence for the reliability and clinical validity of these theoretical constructs will be provided. The method has been described in more detail elsewhere (Horowitz 1997).

Selection of the patterns to be explained sets the stage. Signs, symptoms, maladaptive interpersonal patterns, and irrational identities are usually chosen. Dysfunctional value-appraisals of the self may also be important. Even at this surface level of selecting salient phenomena, it may be possible to infer dynamic associations in terms of what the person desires, fears, or uses to avoid dreaded states. I will illustrate with a case example related to empirical evidence reported elsewhere (Horowitz 1997; Horowitz et al. 1994a).

---

**Table 8–1.** Four steps of configurational formulation

1. Select and describe the phenomena to be explained.
2. Describe states and cycles of the selected phenomena.
3. Identify unresolved themes and indicate the defensive control processes and dysregulation patterns noted in state cycles around these themes.
4. Infer person schemas for each state in terms of role relationship models and, for each theme, the desired, dreaded, and defensive-compromise configurations of role relationship models.

---

*Source.* Adapted from Horowitz 1987, 1997.

### Case Example of Mrs. Sea

Mrs. Patricia Sea was married to James Sea (fictitious names). The Seas lived in relative security and happiness. Unexpectedly, James Sea was violently killed in a robbery. Mrs. Sea was initially in shock and then underwent a period of numbness and depersonalization in which she felt herself going through the motions but not experiencing the vivid sensations of life.

During the ensuing months, Mrs. Sea experienced symptoms of anxiety and depression, with intrusive, unbidden images and pangs of emotion about James. The 1-year anniversary of her husband's death came and went, and she still felt that she had not adequately mourned his loss. She intuitively knew that her mourning was blocked. She felt demoralized. Her symptoms met DSM-III-R (American Psychiatric Association 1987) criteria for major depressive disorder and posttraumatic stress disorder.

## Step 1: Select and Describe Phenomena

A list of salient phenomena regarding Mrs. Sea's complaints and psychiatric symptoms is shown in Table 8–2. The next step in this system of formulation involves the organization of experienced and observed phenomena into states of mind recognized because of the relative co-repetition of the pattern of phenomena.

## Step 2: Describe States and Cycles of States

States can often be defined by describing mood and apparent modulation of emotional medleys and styles of relating to others. It is useful to define states with labels appropriate to the individual patient, although general categorizations may also help clinicians to reach that goal. State definitions found to be empirically valid and clinically useful across patients are shown in Table 8–3.

The personalized descriptions of states of mind for Mrs. Sea are shown in Table 8–4. Once again, now at the state level, the recurrent patterns may be organized into a configuration of desired, dreaded, and compromise states. Such a configuration is shown in Figure 8–1.

| Table 8–2. | A list of phenomena from the case example of Mrs. Sea |
| --- | --- |

**Symptoms**

- Episodes of socially embarrassing, uncontrolled sobbing
- Intrusive images and nightmares related to fantasies of how her husband died
- Pangs of hard-to-describe but negative emotions that felt unbearable if they did not quickly subside
- Trouble sleeping, with fatigue; feeling tense, irritable, and pressured
- Feeling depressed when she "should be happy"

**Signs**

- Generally very descriptive and articulate, but tends to cut off topics related to her reactions to her husband's death
- Usually direct and coherent in discourse, but becomes more vague when talking about a new relationship with a man with whom she may grow more intimate

**Problems in living**

- Takes good care of her children but excessively cloaks them from knowing about their father's death (for example, she did not reveal that there was a gravesite. She avoids going there herself, although she thinks she ought to go and to take her children as well.)
- Loses her temper and feels distress and remorse afterwards

**Unresolved topics**

- Is uncertain about whether to put the death behind her or to confront a grief she feels she has buried in her heart, because were it to emerge, it would overwhelm her physically and emotionally
- Feels conflicted and indecisive about whether to remain independent or to deepen an attractive new intimacy with a man she has begun to date

The general state categories described in Table 8–3 have been found to be reliable in scorings by independent judges of video-taped records of discourse between subjects and clinicians (kappa = .80, agreement 92%). Reliability for individualized state labeling, as illustrated in Table 8–3, has also been demonstrated by independent ratings of ongoing discourse from psychother-apy videotapes (Horowitz et al. 1979). Conflictual topics have been empirically shown to be significantly overrepresented in shimmering and undermodulated states (Horowitz et al. 1993b, 1994a, 1994b).

| **Table 8–3.** Brief definitions of state categories |
| --- |
| **Well-modulated states:**   Relatively smooth flow of expressions without major discordancies between verbal and nonverbal modes. Regardless of intensity, affective displays are expressed with poise. The observer may feel interest and connection. |
| **Overmodulated states:**   Excessive control of expressions: seeming stiff, enclosed, masked, or walled off; affect may appear feigned or false. The observer may feel disconnected. |
| **Undermodulated states:**   Appearance of dysregulation of expressions conveying to observer a sense that the subject is impulsive, uncontrolled, or has intrusive concepts and sharp surges of emotion. The observer may experience surges of emotion as an empathic response, or impulsively want to help the patient regain composure. |
| **Shimmering states:**   Shifting rapidly between undercontrolled emotionality and emotional stifling, or between discordant signs in verbal and nonverbal expressions. The observer may feel uncertain about what is being expressed or the intensity of feeling. |

*Source.*   Adapted from Horowitz et al. 1994.

## Step 3: Identify Unresolved Themes and Defensive Control Processes

Themes are complex sets of beliefs, associational linkages, and potentials for felt emotion. Themes tend to recur in conscious reflection when they are important to the self and when important problems prevent completion of preconscious processes. When a person is engaged in working on unsolved problems, as one hopes is often the case in psychotherapy, the themes of contemplation are likely to contain contradictions in ideas and feelings and conflicts between intentions and motivations.

Anticipating problems and planning how to cope with them is one goal of conscious thought. Conscious contemplation is relatively slow but is a sophisticated tool evolved for effective problem solving. It allows checks and rechecks, albeit at the price of proceeding less quickly than preconscious processing. Solutions that seem apt can be monitored for logic and appraised against alternative solutions. But regulation is necessary when problems and conflicts are intense and difficult. The aim is to keep consciousness from

---

**Table 8–4.** States of mind of Mrs. Sea

**Undermodulated**

- *Intrusive agony of grief:* Experiencing intrusive images and pangs of emotion; feeling ashamed at losing control before others; fearing further flooding with, and being overwhelmed by intensity of, emotion
- *Dull, apathetic depression:* Feeling depleted, disinterested in everything
- *Flare of criticism:* Being too short-tempered with others

**Well modulated**

- *Poignant sorrow:* Feeling sad; experiencing pining and remembrance without losing control
- *Happily excited:* Engaged vivaciously and/or productively; animatedly working

**Overmodulated**

- *Cool and poised:* Feeling numb and floating inside; seeming to be insulated from and remote to others
- *Pressured:* Working hard; being too busy to think

**Shimmering**

- *Struggle with grief:* Experiencing transient tearing or glaring, with momentary stifling of emotional displays or discordancies between verbal and nonverbal signs

---

**Problematic compromise**      **Quasi-adaptive compromise**

| Struggle with grief | Cool and poised |
|---|---|
| Agony of grief | Happily excited |

**Dreaded**                                          **Desired**

**Figure 8–1.** A configuration of states for Mrs. Sea.
*Source.* Adapted from Horowitz 1997.

being flooded with ideational-emotional information that may otherwise lead to jumbled, fragmentary, and confused states of mind.

Defensive control processes influence how a specific theme in a specific context might be attenuated to avoid loss of emotional equilibrium. These processes need not be unitary in operation. Conscious overrides can alter the operation of preconscious modules. Automatic and habitual defensive control processes can sometimes be modified by such overrides. Conscious effort can alter preconscious and defensive-schema–based habits of thinking. New awareness can be repeated, leading to insight and new decisions on how to amend dysfunctional beliefs.

Psychotherapy focuses attention toward such awareness and insight. Creative new syntheses may integrate prior contradictions. Repetitions of new elements and sequences can lead to formation of new beliefs that are then used automatically, without reflective conscious awareness. To repeat, conscious decisions are useful in forming new and linking associations that can integrate competing and incompatible goals.

Defensive control processes can affect preconscious, conscious, and interpersonal processing of meanings. The results may be *adaptive,* regulating information flow to tolerable and hence useful limits for reaching decisions, or *maladaptive,* overregulating emotional information to the point of excessive inhibition of conscious reflective states and thus leaving problematic themes unresolved.

My colleagues and I (Horowitz and Stinson 1991; Horowitz et al. 1992a, 1995b) have used an approach that differentiates purpose and outcome from the cognitive operations that control information processing. Use of this approach leads to a fine-grained classification of defensive control processes in terms of operations that affect the content, form, and organizing principles of communication and thought (Horowitz 1988; Horowitz and Stinson 1995; Horowitz et al. 1990). These defensive control processes are shown in Table 8–5. As described in more detail elsewhere, Mrs. Sea tended to use controls such as those shown in Table 8–6. Her defensive control of self-schemas and role relationship models will be considered below.

---

**Table 8–5.** Defensive control processes

**Content**

1. *Shifting attention*
   Avoids conscious thought, discourse, or action on important unresolved topics by shifting attention to another topic; the shifts may be deliberate (suppression) or may involve less conscious, automatic choices (repression, dissociation, disavowal, or denial).

2. *Juggling concepts about a topic*
   Shifts too often among ideas or emotional valences of ideas, thus preventing a potentially affect-related deepening train of thought; irrelevant details may be amplified. Vital links between ideas and feelings, and between cause and effect, may be obscured.

3. *Sliding meanings and values*
   Adjusts conceptual weighting by minimizing or exaggerating intentions or emotional salience; the resulting appraisal errors and rationalizations may preserve self-esteem or reduce affect ("sweet lemons" or "sour grapes").

4. *Premature disengaging from topics*
   Declares important topics or actions "finished" before reaching closure despite awareness of unresolved dilemmas and contradictions, effectively blocking potentially emotional review of important memories or anticipation of likely future events (e.g., interpersonal tensions).

**Form**

5. *Blocking apt modes of representation*
   Ineffectively represents ideas and feelings about a topic, engaging either in verbal intellectualizations or in preoccupying fantasies. Both can lead to failure to engage in effective action planning. Discourse may lack imagery, metaphors, and clarity, or else may be excessively metaphoric with poor translation of visual images into clear, concrete, meaningful ideas. Both can reduce reactive emotions.

6. *Shifting time span*
   Shifts from most pertinent to alternative, less relevant temporal contexts (e.g., distant past, recent past, here and now, immediate future, distant future) in a manner that avoids or reduces emotionality (e.g., shifts to past memories apparently to avoid confrontation with current relationship difficulties or future jeopardy.

*(continued)*

---

**Table 8–5.**   Defensive control processes *(continued)*

---

7. *Using poor ideational linkage strategies*
   Uses intellectualized analysis of generalities when reflective contemplation or recollection of personalized issues and emotional memories is more appropriate; conversely, may use creatively wide-ranging associations when careful, adaptive planning is more appropriate. The results may be isolated from identity and emotional responses.

8. *Engaging inappropriate arousal levels*
   Shifts to inappropriate level of arousal specifically when addressing a problematic topic; becomes dull, listless, or sleepy or else becomes too excited to do effective contemplation.

**Person schemas**

9. *Shifting self/other roles*
   Abruptly shifts to alternate views of self and other or switches attributes of self and others (projection, role reversal, displacement, compensatory grandiosity, etc.), avoiding dreaded states of fear, shame, rage, and guilt.

10. *Rigidly stabilizing compromise roles*
    Rigidly assumes compromise roles and views of self and other, apparently avoiding desired ones that may have associations with dreaded ones (e.g., wish-fear dilemmas); consequences include avoiding threatening situations and dysphoric emotion, but also withdrawal, numbing, excessive self-preoccupations, and lack of satisfaction.

11. *Altering valuation schemas*
    Shifts to an alternate set of values for appraising self or other with idealizing or devaluating consequences (e.g., unrealistically attributing blame to another, unrealistically criticizing oneself).

---

*Source.*   Adapted from Horowitz 1997.

To a reliable degree, judges of videotapes and transcripts of psychotherapeutic discourse can score both verbal and nonverbal warding-off operations according to well-defined signs of defensive control processes (Horowitz et al. 1993a, 1993b, 1994a, 1995b).

Understanding how a patient uses defensive control processes to shift the set points of information processing can help the psychotherapist assist the patient by suggesting conscious overrides to habitual avoidances or conscious strategies for dealing with episodes of failure to exert adequate control of emotional experience.

**Table 8–6.** Defensive control processes[*] of Mrs. Sea

- Inhibit attention to active memories about James (past) and Sidney (future)
- Facilitate attention to present and near-future tasks not involving intimacy
- Interrupt emotional topics by declarations of "it's over with"
- Retract or obscure lexical communications that lead toward the emotional heart of topics

[*]As used to reduce likelihood of entry into dreaded states of mind.

Once defensive self-concealment, equivocation, and overmodulated states have been reduced and dysregulatory, undermodulated states averted, the patient can work to modify dysfunctional beliefs and erroneous schemas. These conflictual meanings are formulated in the next step.

## Step 4: Construct Role Relationship Models

Schemas include the following aspects of information management: chunking, clustering, listing, outlining, formatting, laying out, generalizing, and smoothing over to organize and connect bits. Schemas can add information and speed, albeit at the cost of introducing erroneous information. Person schemas are enduring schemas that can lead to working models of current relationships. Each interpersonal transaction may undergo parallel preconscious processing until stable working models are achieved. Unconscious fantasies and repertoires of role relationship models may influence these processes, as reviewed by Horowitz and colleagues (Horowitz 1991a; Horowitz et al. 1995a). The same theme, a traumatic memory for example, may be recalled differently in different states, because in each state the processes of construction may affect and be affected by different schemas.

Role relationship models may shift in patterned sequences, and such shifts may be partially responsible for state cycles. Each unit, as run, serves as a stimulus that triggers the activation of the next unit. For example, one may rescue a helpless person, then review the event and feel sadistic for hurting the person in the act of rescue or feel guilty for enjoying the feeling of power experienced during the rescue. To punish oneself for these perceived trans-gressions or to reexperience the heady sensation of power, one may then initiate a repetitive cycle of rescuing others.

Conscious thought and interpersonal communication may evoke active mismatches between discrepant schemas. Such mis-matches lead to alarm emotions (Horowitz 1991a; Horowitz et al. 1992b). Reducing mismatches by forming new schemas or by inte-grating and associating existing schemas can lead to less-alarming rates of escalating emotions. Figure 8–2 illustrates the mismatch of schemas responsible for Mrs. Sea's current conflicts.

An eventual change in schemas, evolved during a process of mourning, can lead to a more controlled emotional state, as shown in Figure 8–3.

Until such reschematization through mourning takes place, Mrs. Sea cannot attain or at least cannot stabilize her desired state, but rather tends to shimmer with or enter into her dreaded state. The role relationship schemas for her desired, dreaded, and com-promise states are shown in Figure 8–4.

Studies of the role relationship model configuration employing independent judges have shown reliability (Eells et al. 1995; Horo-witz and Eells 1993) and predictive validity (Horowitz et al. 1995a) for this construct. Convergent and clinical validity (Horowitz 1989; Horowitz et al. 1991) has also been reported.

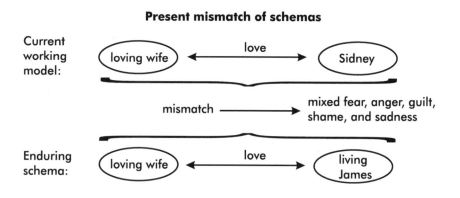

**Present mismatch of schemas**

Current working model:    loving wife ← love → Sidney

mismatch → mixed fear, anger, guilt, shame, and sadness

Enduring schema:    loving wife ← love → living James

**Figure 8–2.**    Present conflict for Mrs. Sea.

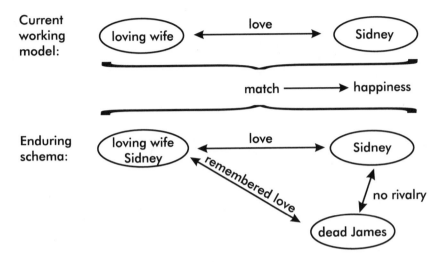

**Figure 8–3.** Future resolution of conflict for Mrs. Sea.

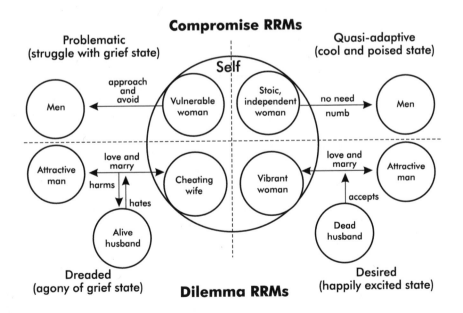

**Figure 8–4.** A role relationship model (RRM) configuration for Mrs. Sea.

# Planning Therapy

Psychotherapists can use an understanding gained from such formulations and a knowledge of likely processes of change to plan clinical technique. State-stabilizing interventions can be planned once state cycles have been observed. Therapists can encourage patients to use conscious overrides to habitual unconscious defensive control processes. Contradictory beliefs can then be addressed and new integrations developed.

Work in therapy can "unpack" the complex meanings that lead into highly emotional states. Configurations and state cycles can be gradually understood by identifying conflicts between different role relationship models. Some techniques may involve attention, focusing, and priming to activate adaptive role relationship models and deactivate maladaptive ones. For example, the therapist may clarify specific representations of incomplete, bad, strange, and evil self-schemas and thereby help the patient to de-center him- or herself from these attributions. Or the therapist may bolster and center the patient's attention on competent/realistic and current self-schemas by heightening concepts and slowing down contemplation to increase rational constructs and cause-and-effect reasoning. The patient may be encouraged to plan new and possibly more adaptive behaviors and to repeat these. Such repetition helps the patient to develop new script schemas and new defensive schemas slowly over time, as seems necessary for eventual automatic functioning.

Usually warded-off but motivationally important relationship models can lead to transference reactions. Interpreting these reactions can assist in explicating motives for repeated maladaptive interpersonal behavioral patterns that lead to distress. Such interpretation also clarifies usually warded-off goals and emotions and the reasons for defensive avoidances.

Countertransference can also be formulated in a helpful way. Patients often maneuver the therapist into their own wish/fear dilemmas and then watch to see how the therapist handles that plight. If they like the therapist's solution, they identify with it. The use of person schemas may help beginning therapists to deal with such role-reversals so that patients may have time to form new roles for themselves. After this purpose has been served, the therapist may then interpret these reversals if they become defensive avoidances.

# Summary

Phenomena vary by state. Motivation can be inferred by examining cycles of states that recur in maladaptive cycles. Some states are compromises and result from defensive control processes, whereas others are closer to the individual's most desired or feared feelings. Individuals may have multiple self-schemas and role relationship models that lead to these different states. Units in these repertoires of organized meaning may be shifted by modifying the set point of defensive control processes. Changes in defenses, according to habitual defensive schemas, can lead to a state cycle. Thus, state cycles are due partially to both sequences of role relationship models and defensive scripts for shifting these person schemas.

Formulating in terms of four levels—phenomena, states and state cycles, defensive control processes, and role relationship models—can help clinicians clarify complex state variations in symptoms, explain why state cycles occur, and provide a basis for planing how to intervene.

# References

American Psychiatric Association: Diagnostic and Statistical Manual of Mental Disorders, 3rd Edition, Revised. Washington, DC, American Psychiatric Association, 1987

American Psychiatric Association: Diagnostic and Statistical Manual of Mental Disorders, 4th Edition. Washington, DC, American Psychiatric Association, 1994

Eells TD, Horowitz MJ, Singer J, et al: The role relationship models method: a comparison of independently derived case formulations. Psychotherapy Research 5:161–175, 1995

Horowitz MJ: States of Mind: Configurational Analysis of Individual Personality, 2nd Edition. New York, Plenum, 1987

Horowitz MJ: Unconsciously determined defensive strategies, in Psychodynamics and Cognition. Edited by Horowitz MJ. Chicago, IL, University of Chicago Press, 1988, pp 49–80

Horowitz MJ: Relationship schema formulation: role-relationship models and intrapsychic conflict. Psychiatry 52:260–274, 1989

Horowitz MJ: Person schemas, in Person Schemas and Maladaptive Interpersonal Patterns. Edited by Horowitz MJ. Chicago, IL, University of Chicago Press, 1991a, pp 13–31

Horowitz MJ: States, schemas, and control: general theories for psychotherapy integration. Journal of Psychotherapy Integration 1:85–102, 1991b

Horowitz MJ: Formulation as a Basis for Planning Psychotherapy Treatment. Washington, DC, American Psychiatric Press, 1997

Horowitz MJ, Eells TD: Case formulations using role-relationship model configurations: a reliability study. Psychotherapy Research 3:57–68, 1993

Horowitz MJ, Stinson CH: University of California at San Francisco, Center for the Study of Neuroses, Program on Conscious and Unconscious Mental Processes, in Psychotherapy Research: An International Review of Programmatic Studies. Edited by Beutler LE, Crago M. Washington, DC American Psychological Association, 1991, pp 107–114

Horowitz MJ, Stinson CH: Consciousness and processes of control. Journal of Psychotherapy Practice and Research 4:123–139, 1995

Horowitz MJ, Marmar C, Wilner N: Analysis of patient states and state transitions. J Nerv Ment Dis 167:91–99, 1979

Horowitz MJ, Markman HC, Stinson CH, et al: A classification theory of defense, in Repression and Dissociation: Implications for Personality Theory, Psychopathology, and Health. Edited by Singer J. Chicago, IL, University of Chicago Press, 1990, pp 61–84

Horowitz MJ, Luborsky L, Popp C: A comparison of the role-relationship models configuration and the core conflictual relationship theme, in Person Schemas and Maladaptive Interpersonal Patterns. Edited by Horowitz MJ. Chicago, IL, University of Chicago Press, 1991, pp 213–220

Horowitz MJ, Cooper S, Fridhandler B, et al: Control processes and defense mechanisms. Journal of Psychotherapy Practice and Research 1:324–336, 1992a

Horowitz MJ, Fridhandler BF, Stinson CH: Person schemas and emotion, in Psychoanalytic Perspectives. Edited by Shapiro T, Emde RN. New York, International Universities Press, 1992b, pp 173–208

Horowitz MJ, Milbrath C, Reidbord S, et al: Elaboration and dyselaboration: measures of expression and defense in discourse. Psychotherapy Research 3:278–293, 1993a

Horowitz MJ, Stinson C, Curtis D, et al: Topics and signs: defensive control of emotional expression. J Consult Clin Psychol 61:421–430, 1993b

Horowitz MJ, Milbrath C, Ewert M, et al: Cyclical patterns of states of mind in psychotherapy. Am J Psychiatry 151:1767–1770, 1994a

Horowitz MJ, Milbrath C, Jordan DS, et al: Expressive and defensive behavior during discourse on unresolved topics: a single case study. J Pers 62:527–563, 1994b

Horowitz MJ, Eells T, Singer J, et al: Role relationship models for case formulation. Arch Gen Psychiatry 53:627–656, 1995a

Horowitz MJ, Znoj H, Stinson C: Defensive control processes: use of theory in research, formulation, and therapy of stress response syndromes, in Handbook of Coping. Edited by Zeidner M, Endler N. New York, Wiley, 1995b, pp 532–553

# Index

*Page numbers printed in **boldface** type refer to tables or figures.*